SECRETS OF
YOGA

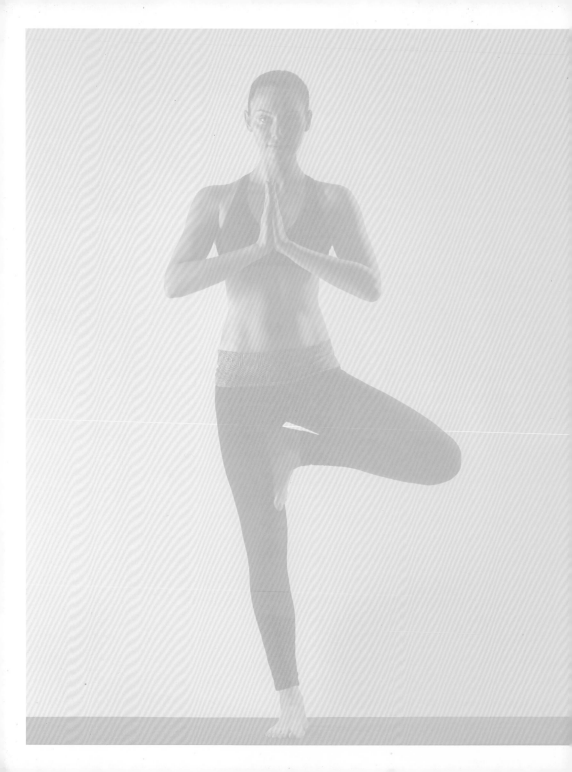

SECRETS OF
YOGA

JENNIE BITTLESTON

IVY PRESS

This edition published in the UK and North America in 2017 by
Ivy Press
An imprint of The Quarto Group
The Old Brewery, 6 Blundell Street
London N7 9BH, United Kingdom
T (0)20 7700 6700 F (0)20 7700 8066
www.QuartoKnows.com

First published in 2000

British Library Cataloguing-in-Publication Data
A catalogue record for this book is available from the British Library

ISBN: 978-1-78240-464-4

Text by Helen Varley

This book was conceived, designed and produced by
Ivy Press
58 West Street, Brighton BN1 2RA, United Kingdom

Art Director: Peter Bridgewater
Editorial Director: Sophie Collins
Designers: Kevin Knight, Jane Lanaway and Ginny Zeal
Project Editor: Caroline Earle
Picture Researcher: Liz Eddison
Photographer: Guy Ryecart
Illustrations: Coral Mula, Michael Courtney and Andrew Milne
Three-dimensional models: Mark Jamieson
Editorial Assistant: Jenny Campbell

Printed in China

10 9 8 7 6 5 4 3 2

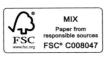

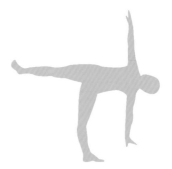

Note from the publisher Information given in this book is
not intended to be taken as a replacement for medical advice.
Any person with a condition requiring medical attention should
consult a qualified medical practitioner or therapist.

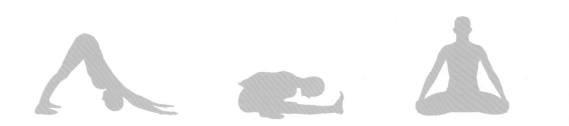

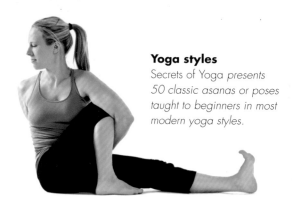

Yoga styles
*Secrets of Yoga presents
50 classic asanas or poses
taught to beginners in most
modern yoga styles.*

HOW TO USE THIS BOOK

Secrets of Yoga is a startup guide for anyone just beginning yoga, and a useful handbook for teachers and for more experienced students who wish to practice between classes. Chapter 1 traces the evolution of yoga, Chapter 2 looks at the basics, and Chapter 3 takes you through your very first practice. Chapter 4 presents 40 classic poses roughly in the order in which you would normally learn them and Chapter 5 completes your introduction to yoga by explaining how to create a program for home practice.

Levels of Difficulty

Within each category the poses appear in order of increasing complexity, and each has an icon

 BEGINNERS for complete beginners

 INTERMEDIATE slightly more advanced—you have worked through Chapter 3 at least once

 ADVANCED more advanced poses to use when your body has gained some flexibility

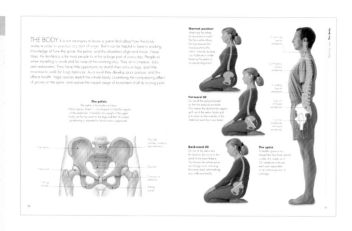

Basic information
The first part looks at what you need to begin, the body and breathing, and how to approach the poses.

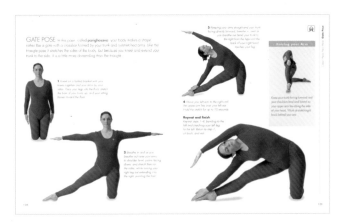

Poses

Full-color pages show each pose in detail, with a clear introduction explaining the name and the purpose of the pose and its health-giving benefits. Numbered illustrations and captions show how to achieve the pose step-by-step.

Analysis

Black-and-white pages analyze each pose. The main text explores the pose, while the correct positioning of each body part is pinpointed with annotation and arrows show direction of stretching.

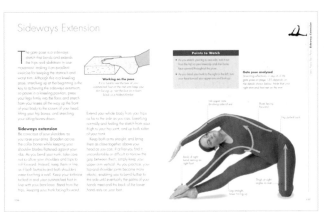

Home practice

The book finishes with three sample programs based on the 50 classic poses presented in Chapters 3 and 4.

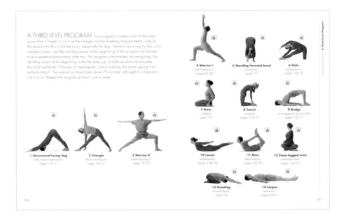

Why Yoga?

Of the many fitness systems popular today, yoga is the oldest, yet the multiplicity of classes and courses available all over the world testify to the 21st-century relevance of this ancient art. Its roots are buried more than 4,000 years deep in the soil of southern Asia, and as it has grown, the great tree of yoga has developed many branches. Yoga is meditation and it is philosophy, it is chanting and deep, rhythmic breathing, and it is healing through exercise.

Restoring harmony

"Union" is the meaning of the word "yoga," and in this increasingly fragmented age yoga offers a way of restoring harmony. It teaches how to unite body and mind, and mind and spirit. It brings physical fitness and increased energy, and a feeling of well-being. It offers relaxation and calm to counter the anxiety and mental stress of 21st-century living. It replaces mood swings and emotional strain with a balanced mind and clear thinking.

This book is for newcomers to yoga, for anyone—from teenagers to the over-

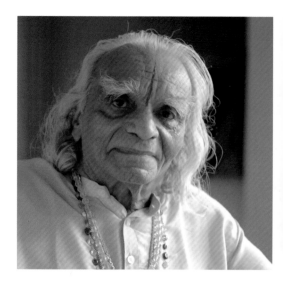

Contemporary teachers
The popularity of Iyengar yoga, founded in the 20th century by the Indian teacher, B.K.S. Iyengar (1918–2014), testifies to yoga's importance to the modern world.

nineties—who is interested in learning yoga or just beginning. It has been written for anyone intending to learn alone at home, and as a useful handbook for practice between classes. As well as explaining the basics—the classic and modern styles, when, where, and how to practice—it focuses on 50 classic poses practiced in the traditional schools of yoga and in the modern styles which derive from them.

Caution

If you are taking medication, have recently had an operation, have a chronic complaint or a recent injury, or if your mobility is restricted, check with a doctor or a physical therapist before beginning. Always learn with an experienced instructor who knows about your condition.

- Do not practice standing poses if you have high blood pressure or heart disease.

- Do not practice sitting poses if you have had a hip replacement.

- Do not practice forward bends, side bending, or twisting movements of the trunk if you have a back injury or a prolapsed intervertebral disk.

- Do not practice shoulder stands or inverted poses if you are menstruating or have dizzy spells; eye, ear or sinus problems; a head, neck, or back injury; high blood pressure; or migraines.

- Never adopt a position that causes any pain or undue discomfort since you risk injury.

- Do not practice backbends if you have heart disease or high blood pressure, or a slipped disk or other back problems.

- If you have a knee injury, do not practice kneeling poses or backbends.

- If you have osteoporosis or a stiff back, ease very gently into stretches and twists and do not attempt backbends, inverted poses, or the boat or half-boat.

- Do not begin yoga during pregnancy.

STYLES & SCHOOLS

The evolution of yoga is believed to span almost 4,000 years, and during this long development it has branched into many different schools. Some concentrate on the mind and meditation, some on exercise and breathing. This chapter maps the story of yoga, from its origins in the Indian subcontinent some 4,000 years ago to its spread worldwide during the 20th century. It introduces some yoga luminaries of the past whose writings and observations inspired the great classic schools. And it ends by focusing on some key 20th-century teachers who founded styles and schools that are carrying yoga forward into its fifth millennium.

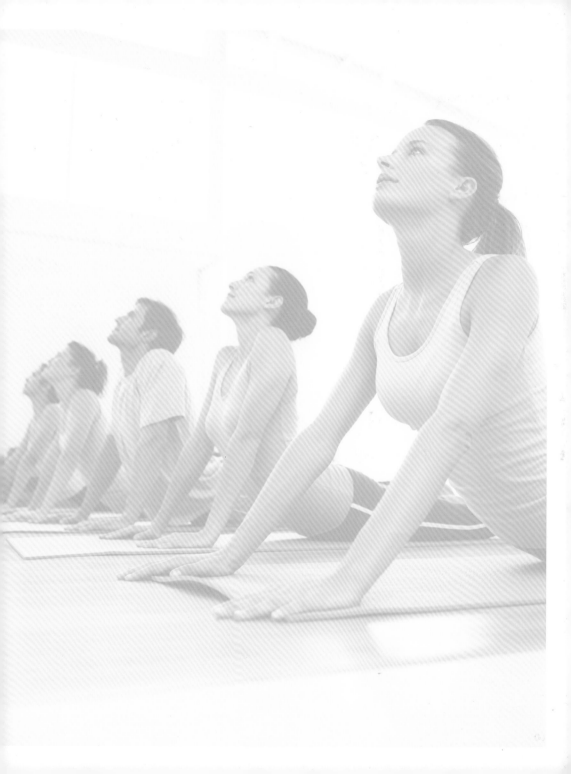

The Philosophy of Yoga

In the West, most people think of yoga as a system of exercises designed to maintain health and prevent illness. But although physical exercise is indeed important, yoga practice synthesizes body, mind, and spirit. Thought is a major component of yoga practice.

Yoga evolved primarily as a philosophy; the exercises or "asanas" developed later as a way of concentrating the mind in order to be able to meditate more deeply. The ultimate aim of yoga has always been to achieve oneness with what some call universal thought or consciousness, and others call God. Today, meditation is still an integral part of practice in many schools and styles of yoga, while in others it is considered an advanced technique and not taught to beginners.

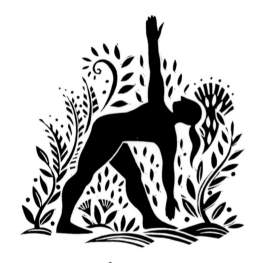

Awareness
Yoga emphasizes opening oneself up to the influences of nature and the natural world.

The way of yoga

Yoga is not a religion, but its continued development has been influenced by the ideas of many great thinkers and teachers. Their writings provide a set of commonsense principles by which to live a peaceful and healthy life. Foremost among their collective beliefs is the principle of nonviolence. Yoga works to establish inner peace and mental and physical harmony.

The path of yoga is a personal search for deeper self-knowledge through the asanas or poses, and through breathing, relaxation, and learning to quiet and focus the mind. The way of yoga is a spiritual journey into the self and beyond.

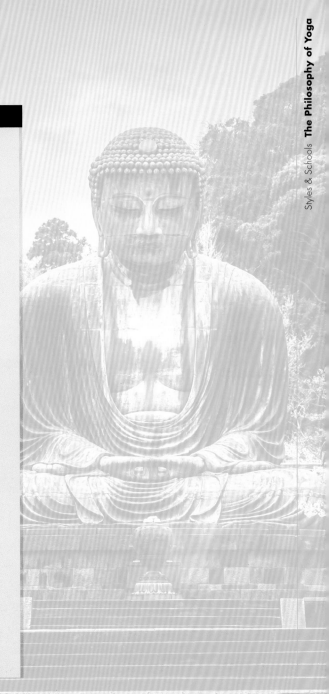

Rules for Right Living

The sage Patañjali who lived some 2,000 years ago left a collection of writings called the *Yoga Sutras* (a sutra is a short saying, packed with meaning). They contain simple advice for living a useful and fulfilling life. Here are ten of his best-known guidelines:

THE FIVE YAMAS
—or how to be kind to others

1 Refrain from violence in thought, word, and deed.

2 Do not steal.

3 Do not covet the possessions and achievements of others.

4 Speak and live the truth.

5 Practice self-restraint and refrain from indulging in excess and sexual depravity.

THE FIVE NIYAMAS
—or how to be kind to yourself

1 Maintain mental purity and physical cleanliness.

2 Rise above objects of desire.

3 Accept your situation in life.

4 Repeat the sacred words of the great teachers.

5 Devote yourself to a personal deity— or the universal consciousness.

Buddha
Gautama Buddha is sometimes described as the first yogi.

ANCIENT ART
The origins of yoga are buried in ancient history. Historians think that the ideas from which it evolved may have emerged in southwestern Asia more than 4,000 years ago, and been carried southward through the Indian subcontinent by migrating tribes. Artifacts unearthed in excavations of the ancient Indus Valley civilizations, which flourished around 1500 BCE, show people meditating. The Upanishads, written between 900 and 400 BCE, are the oldest known writings on yoga.

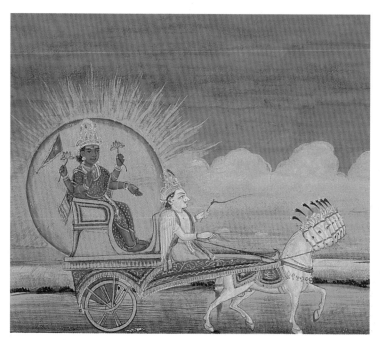

Karma yoga
The Bhagavad Gita (Song of the Lord), a gripping epic tale of a battle between two clans, was written around 300 BCE It presented karma yoga, a new yoga of selfless action that explores ways of dealing with life's many problems.

Buddha's birthplace

The Himalayan foothills were the birthplace of Gautama Buddha around 550 BCE, a time of religious and intellectual ferment in the East. He became a wandering sage who followed the path of raja yoga to attain enlightenment.

Lotus pose

The ancient sages were often depicted meditating in the cross-legged lotus pose or padmasana, a passive sitting position which, once mastered, is comfortable and frees the mind to concentrate.

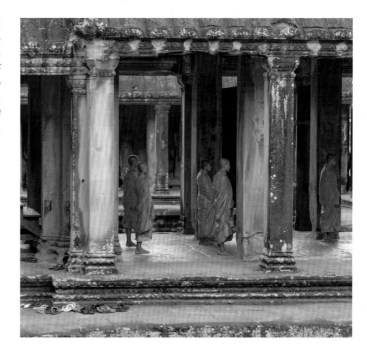

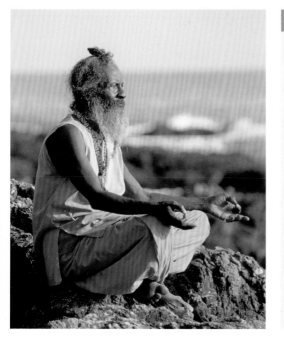

Raja Yoga

The earliest form of yoga was meditation. In the art of the ancient East the Buddha was often depicted meditating, his knees crossed in one of the classic cross-legged sitting positions. These were the first asanas or yoga postures, developed by the sages because they enabled them to sit in meditation without moving for long periods. The ancient form of yoga Buddha practiced survives today as raja yoga—"the king of yogas"—because all yoga pathways are said to lead to it. Raja yoga is the way of deep meditation. Through it, dedicated individuals and communities of yogis explore the realm of abstract thought, seeking to tap into universal consciousness, to attain spiritual unity with the universe through a life dedicated to yoga.

Classic Schools

The tree of yoga has many great branches, for along with the countless thousands of people who practice the exercise-based styles of modern yoga, there are numerous followers of the great classic schools that arose in ancient times. Most of these evolved during the first millennium BCE, when freethinkers broke away from the religious establishment of the Indian subcontinent to develop new philosophies and ascetic ways of living.

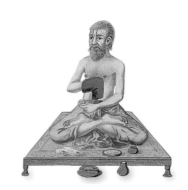

Kapila
This sage, who lived about 2,750 years ago, founded the samkhya philosophy, which contributed concepts such as life force and life energy to yoga.

BEFORE **1000** BCE	c. **900** BCE	c. **500** BCE	c. **300** BCE
RAJA YOGA	**JNANA YOGA**	Gautama Buddha and his followers practice the ancient meditation techniques of raja yoga, and achieve the state of nirvana or loss of the Self in a universal oneness.	**KARMA YOGA**
The practice of meditating sitting in a cross-legged position reaches the Indian subcontinent from Persia, and is carried southward by Dravidian-speaking people. Raja yoga, "the king of yoga," is practiced by philosophers seeking spiritual unity with universal knowledge or consciousness.	Philosophers exploring intuitive knowledge develop the yoga of wisdom or jnana ("geeyana") yoga. Their ideas appear in the Upanishads, a set of innovative scriptures that contain the first written accounts of yogic practice and experience. Jnana yoga develops intuitive knowledge through meditation.		The sage Vyasa writes the *Bhagavad Gita* (*Song of the Lord*), introducing a yoga of action, karma yoga, as a conversation on the eve of the battle between Arjuna, a warrior chief, and his charioteer, the god Krishna. Karma yoga emphasizes taking the right action at the right time to avoid future unhappiness.

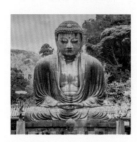

BUDDHA

The last great classic school

The first millennium CE saw the development of new meditational practices. These included chanting incantations or mantras, such as "om," and contemplating geometric patterns called mandalas. From this new wave of breakaway thinking emerged hatha yoga (pronounced "hatta"), the last great classic yoga school. "Ha" means "sun" and "tha" means "moon" and the name refers to breathing exercises called pranayama, which are practiced as a way of linking mind and body. Hatha yoga was the first school that combined physical exercises and deep breathing to help concentrate the mind for meditation. During the 1400s, a sage called Swami Svatmarama produced a work known as the *Hathapradipika* (*The Compendium of Hatha Yoga*), which is believed to be the first written guide to hatha yoga.

c. **200** BCE	c. **300**S CE	c. **1000–1200** CE	c. **1000** CE
The sage Patañjali writes the *Yoga Sutras*, giving guidelines on meditation and the practice of yoga—the first yoga manual.	**TANTRIC YOGA** Asanga, a Buddhist philosopher, initiates tantric philosophy, incorporating yoga ideas and practices, in which the senses and the imagination are harnessed to attain ecstatic states, which may lead to enlightenment. It encourages mantra yoga—chanting sacred words—to aid meditation.	**BHAKTI YOGA** The sage Ramanuja initiates bhakti yoga, the yoga of devotion to a personal god. He teaches devotion to a supreme Brahman, creator of the universe, a loving and understanding presence. Through service to God or to other people, through prayer, and through faith, one achieves enlightenment.	**HATHA YOGA** The development of physical exercises during the tantric era paved the way for hatha yoga. It was the first school to recognize asanas, breathing and cleansing exercises, and visualization techniques as valid aids to attaining union with universal consciousness through meditation.

PATAÑJALI

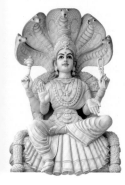

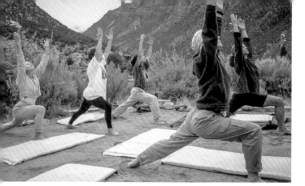

Yoga reaches out
During the 20th century the tree of yoga spread its canopy across the Western world.

CONTEMPORARY STYLES

The latest chapter in the story of yoga began in the 1800s, when explorers, academics, soldiers, and administrators from the West who resided in India translated the ancient yoga texts and studied the asanas. By 1900, yogis from India were touring the West and in the mid-1900s, Paramahansa Yogananda, author of the well-known *Autobiography of a Yogi*, settled in the US. Hatha yoga was the classic school destined to influence the modern world, since its emphasis on asanas, breathing, and healing appealed to the Western mind. After World War II many Westerners visited India to study hatha yoga, and respected Indian teachers, most notably B.K.S. Iyengar, taught in the West.

Iyengar
B.K.S. Iyengar married classic hatha yoga with detailed Western knowledge of the body to establish a new yoga style based on accurate positioning and movement.

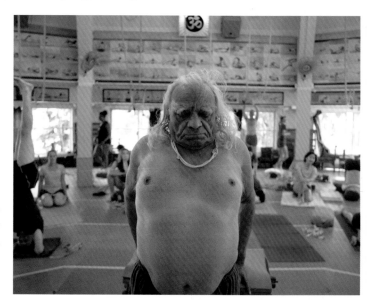

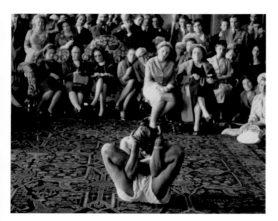

Pioneer

The teaching of yoga to mixed groups of men and women students in India was pioneered by B.K.S. Iyengar during the 1940s. Iyengar developed his own style of yoga and founded the Iyengar Institute in Poona. Today it has branches in many Western countries.

1893: Vivekenada takes yoga to North America

1800s: Europeans translate ancient yoga texts

c. 500 CE: Yoga reaches Tibet, China, and Japan

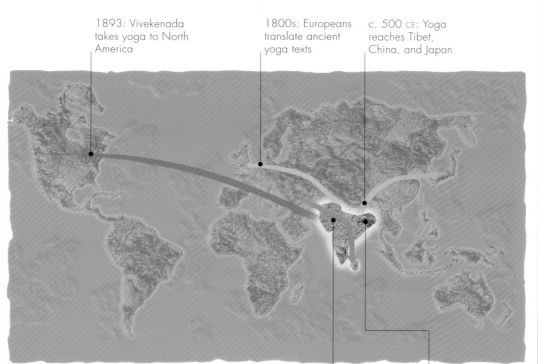

The spread of yoga

In modern times yoga has spread eastward beyond the Indian subcontinent, and out to the West. Today, its popularity worldwide proves its relevance to pressurized 21st-century living.

c. 1000 CE: Hatha yoga founded in Northern India

c. 300s CE: Tantric yoga schools emerge in NE India

Yoga for the 21st Century

Yoga originated as a healing art, whose purpose was to dispel disharmonies of mind and body that might impede an individual's journey along the path to universal wholeness and understanding. Such disharmonies might express themselves in rigidities of the body or in physical illness, and in discontent or anxiety. Over the centuries, yoga sages discovered how to calm and overcome them by gentle stretching and exercise, by slow, rhythmic breathing, which gradually quiets the mind, and by techniques such as visualization and meditation, which concentrate the mind.

Mental healing
Yoga gently erodes the mental turmoil of 21st-century living, bringing peace and personal fulfillment.

Modern appeal

Today, just as in ancient times, people neglect their bodies, injure themselves, and develop illnesses. They become dissatisfied, agitated, and unhappy. Yoga continues to be relevant because it provides some answers to the difficulties of living in the modern world. The styles and schools of yoga that are popular today are those which, like Iyengar yoga, focus on stretching and movement. We sit for most of the day when traveling, at work, as well as when relaxing, yet if bones, joints, and muscles are not stretched and moved,

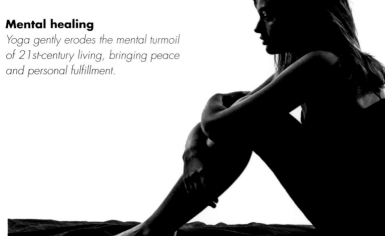

the body deteriorates. Yoga restores natural flexibility to stiff backs, necks, and limbs. It helps the body heal after strain and trauma, and practiced regularly, it promotes health and prevents illness.

People everywhere react against the speed of contemporary living, against the unquestioning acceptance of competition in everyday life, and against the effects of overcrowding. Many people turn to yoga as a remedy for the effects of stress on mind and body. Experiments in the US at the Menninger Institute and at other respected medical research centers have shown that by a combination of breathing, visualization, and concentration, yogis can reduce their heart rate and blood pressure.

Yoga is a holistic practice, not just an exercise system. When you begin yoga, you harness the powers of the body and the mind to soothe the nerves and calm the body systems, reducing stress and allowing the body to restore normal function. Rhythmic breathing, called pranayama, and meditation techniques enhance this healing process. They are an important part of hatha yoga, and in Iyengar yoga, pranayama and concentration techniques are taught to advanced students.

PRACTICING
YOGA

In contrast with most of the exercise systems that have become fashionable in recent years, yoga is a minimalist art, requiring almost no expense or preparation. Your own body is all the equipment you really need. There is no special clothing to buy or equipment to use, and you can practice almost anywhere. This chapter explains the basics: when to practice, how often, and for how long; the parts of the body that need special attention, and the essentials of breathing and relaxation. But yoga is a holistic art, involving the mind as much as the body, and the chapter ends by explaining how yoga might deepen your understanding of your mind and your personality, and lead you to explore its hidden spiritual dimension.

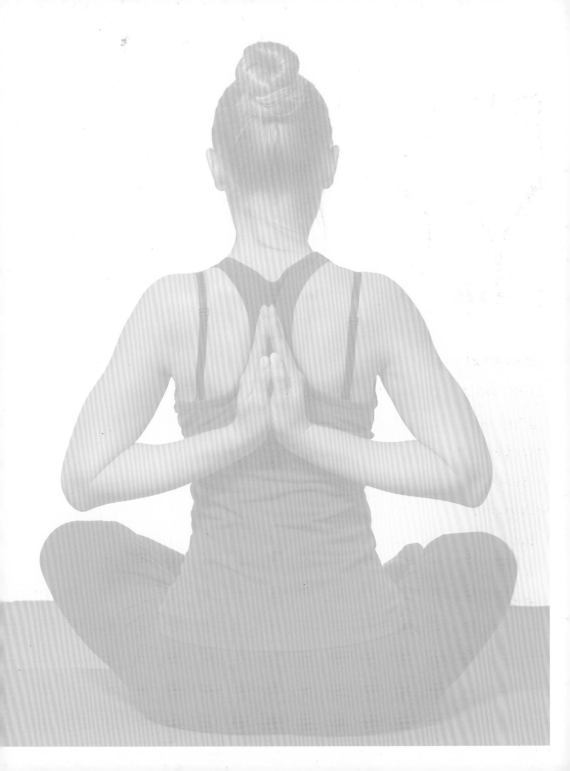

Preparation

If you are just beginning yoga, learning alone at home, or needing a place to work on poses between classes, you must find a place where you will be able to stretch with a minimum of interruption. It may be tempting to practice outdoors if the weather is warm, but it is not advisable to practice yoga in the hot sun, and there can be distractions from traffic and building work. It can be hard to find a place at home where you can be undisturbed by telephones, doorbells, or family members, but think of using your bedroom, a bathroom, a utility room, an office, or a den. Put a "do not disturb" notice on the door.

Aids to practice
Ideally, choose a fairly empty room for your practice. You need enough floor space in all directions, a free length of wall, and the items shown here.

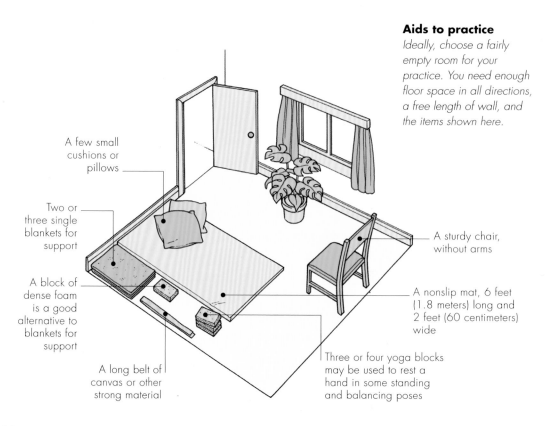

A few small cushions or pillows

Two or three single blankets for support

A block of dense foam is a good alternative to blankets for support

A long belt of canvas or other strong material

A sturdy chair, without arms

A nonslip mat, 6 feet (1.8 meters) long and 2 feet (60 centimeters) wide

Three or four yoga blocks may be used to rest a hand in some standing and balancing poses

Making time

Practice as often as you like, but practice regularly. Do not be overambitious at first. It is best to set aside a certain time on a certain day a week to practice and be disciplined about keeping that weekly date. Allow for half an hour at first, working up to longer sessions as you are able. Some people like to practice for a short time every day, early in the morning, or before bed, and to have one longer session once a week.

Yoga imposes very few rules, and some poses aid digestion—for example, you can practice the hero floor pose straight after eating a meal. This is not true of most poses, however, so as a rule of thumb, do not practice for four hours after a large meal or two hours after a snack.

For yoga, wear comfortable clothes that stretch easily, such as a t-shirt and leggings, a leotard, or jogging pants and a sweatshirt. Practice barefoot. If your hair is long it is best to fasten it up so it cannot obscure your vision.

THE BODY

It is not necessary to know a great deal about how the body works in order to practice any style of yoga. But it can be helpful to have a working knowledge of how the spine, the pelvis, and the shoulders align and move. These days, the tendency is for most people to sit for a large part of every day. People sit when traveling to work and for most of the working day. They sit in cinemas, bars, and restaurants. They have little opportunity to stretch their arms or legs, and little incentive to walk for long distances. As a result they develop poor posture, and this affects health. Yoga asanas stretch the whole body, countering the compressing effect of gravity on the spine, and restore the natural range of movement of all its moving parts.

The pelvis

The pelvis is the body's linchpin.
"Pelvis" means "basin" — it is shaped to hold the organs
of the abdomen. It transfers the weight of the upper
body via the hip joints to the legs and feet. Its proper
positioning is essential to almost every yoga pose.

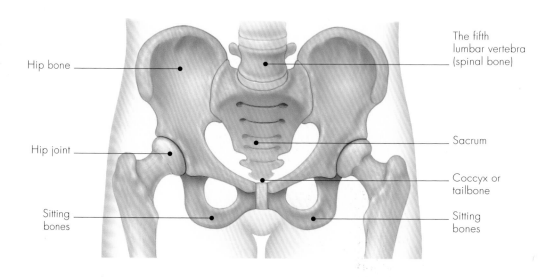

Hip bone

Hip joint

Sitting bones

The fifth lumbar vertebra (spinal bone)

Sacrum

Coccyx or tailbone

Sitting bones

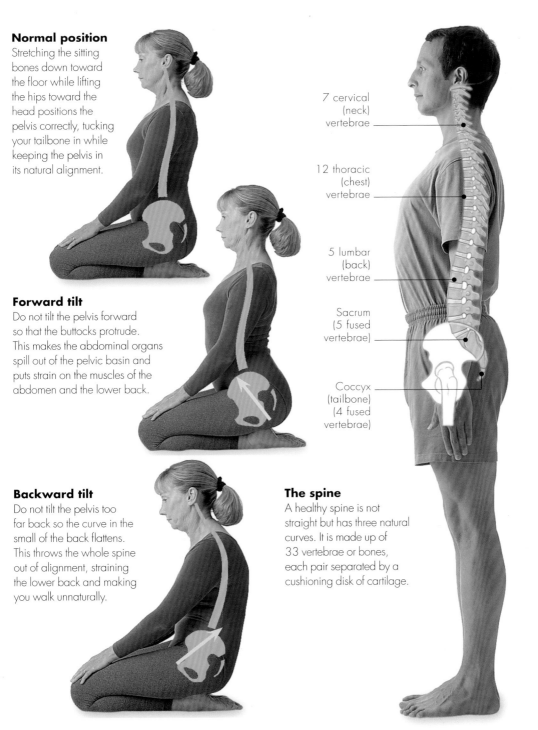

Normal position

Stretching the sitting bones down toward the floor while lifting the hips toward the head positions the pelvis correctly, tucking your tailbone in while keeping the pelvis in its natural alignment.

Forward tilt

Do not tilt the pelvis forward so that the buttocks protrude. This makes the abdominal organs spill out of the pelvic basin and puts strain on the muscles of the abdomen and the lower back.

Backward tilt

Do not tilt the pelvis too far back so the curve in the small of the back flattens. This throws the whole spine out of alignment, straining the lower back and making you walk unnaturally.

7 cervical (neck) vertebrae

12 thoracic (chest) vertebrae

5 lumbar (back) vertebrae

Sacrum (5 fused vertebrae)

Coccyx (tailbone) (4 fused vertebrae)

The spine

A healthy spine is not straight but has three natural curves. It is made up of 33 vertebrae or bones, each pair separated by a cushioning disk of cartilage.

27

Breathing & Relaxation

Breathing is both a physical and a mental process, a link between body and mind. Breathing at a normal pace supplies the blood with oxygen and other nutrients, and these keep the body and brain functioning. Rapid breathing or hyperventilation reduces the supply of oxygen to the brain, causing dizziness and abnormal heart rhythm, tension, panic, and black-outs. Slowing the breathing and restoring its natural rhythm restores calm and normal functioning.

Good breathing habits

Remembering to breathe properly is an important part of every pose. In the early stages, the focus is on developing good breathing habits. People living a pressured existence often develop shallow breathing habits as a stress response. Yoga discourages that tendency, helping to reestablish normal breathing patterns.

The guidelines on how to perform the asanas contain frequent reminders to "breathe normally." This may seem obvious, but when trying to concentrate on a movement it can seem almost natural to hold your breath, and you need to watch for those moments. If your nasal passages are blocked because of a cold or other sinus problem you will have to breathe through the mouth, but normally, you should breathe through the nose.

Some instructions about when to breathe in and when to breathe out are

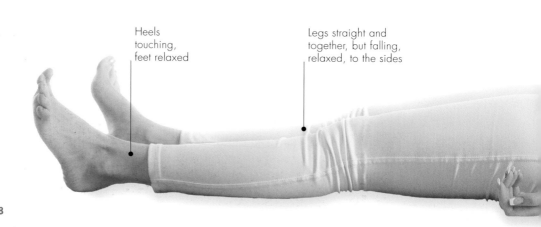

Heels touching, feet relaxed

Legs straight and together, but falling, relaxed, to the sides

given in the captions explaining each pose. In general, you breathe out on an exertion—as you lift or bend forward, for example. Breathe in, breathe out as you execute the movement, then breathe normally again.

Breathing & relaxation

Stretching and rhythmic breathing relax body and mind. Relaxation is an essential part of yoga. A practice session should begin with a few moments of repose in a restful posture—sitting in a simple cross-legged pose, for example, and the more demanding poses should be followed by a few brief moments of rest just standing, kneeling, or lying down, until your natural breathing rhythm has been restored.

Corpse pose
Savasana I, analyzed in detail on pages 64–65, helps relax body and mind during moments of particular stress and tension.

Arms resting a few inches from the sides of the body, palms turned up

Head in line with body

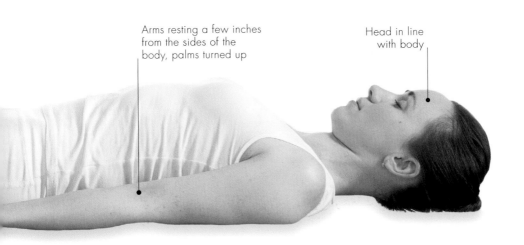

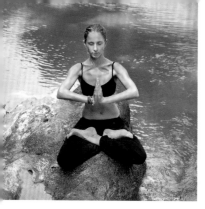

Spiritual union
The word "yoga" signifies spiritual union between the individual and the world beyond the self.

MIND & SPIRIT
Learning to perform the asanas and regulate your breathing are ways of learning to calm and focus your mind. Mastering these skills helps you progress. Concentration is the ability to focus on a particular thought or action. Yoga directs your attention to something physical: a posture, and for a short time this holds your attention. In this way you exercise and improve your concentration. One of the greatest problems people have in everyday life is being able to concentrate, and yoga can be a great help. Moreover, achieving the ability to concentrate is the first step on the path to exploring the spiritual dimension of yoga by bringing meditation into your life. Meditation is total concentration.

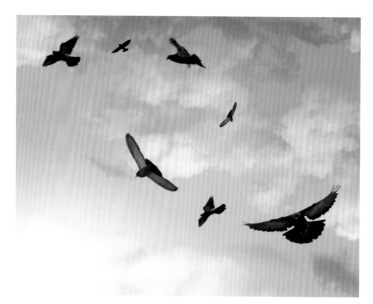

Free spirit
The ultimate aim of yoga is to release the mind from the restrictions of the physical body and allow the spirit to explore new levels of consciousness.

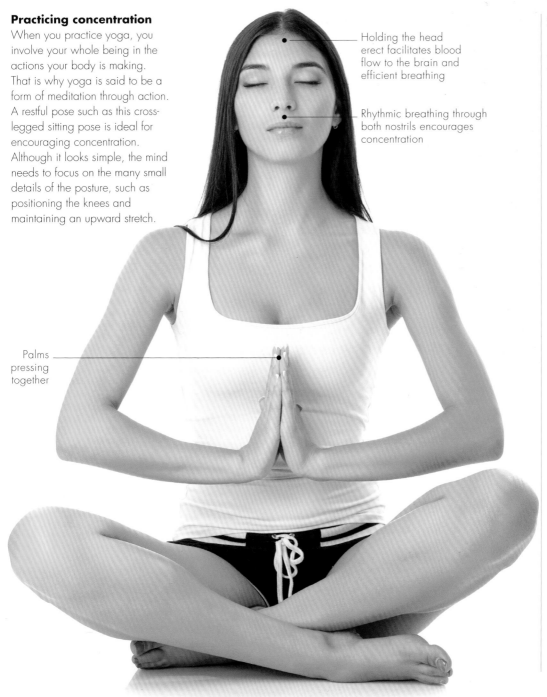

Practicing concentration

When you practice yoga, you involve your whole being in the actions your body is making. That is why yoga is said to be a form of meditation through action. A restful pose such as this cross-legged sitting pose is ideal for encouraging concentration. Although it looks simple, the mind needs to focus on the many small details of the posture, such as positioning the knees and maintaining an upward stretch.

Holding the head erect facilitates blood flow to the brain and efficient breathing

Rhythmic breathing through both nostrils encourages concentration

Palms pressing together

Emotion & Control

To practice yoga is to make some quiet space in your life, a little time to let negative emotions subside, and allow the natural rhythms of mind and body to reassert themselves. Rather than give inner turmoil opportunities to express itself in sudden or violent outbursts, yoga gives strong emotions gentle physical release through intense stretching, and deflects the mind away from them by directing the attention on precise movement and accurate positioning. The result is the diffusion of anger and resentment, the lifting of heavy spirits, and the calming and containing of hurt and mental discomfort. At the end of a concentrated yoga practice, feelings of ease and tranquillity saturate both the body and mind.

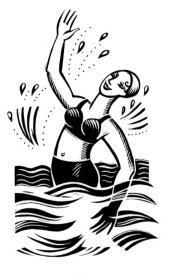

Enrichment
Yoga enriches your inner life, teaching you to be less dependent on outside events for happiness.

Tranquillity

The ability to restore tranquillity to mind and body is a major gift of yoga to an increasingly turbulent world. People regularly have to deal with mounting stress in all aspects of their lives. In time, many succumb to the emotional turmoil this causes, and this can result in clinical depression, the breakdown of relationships, and, more and more frequently, aggressive outbursts, such as road rage, and rising crime rates. A tranquil person radiating inner harmony benefits others by transmitting calm and reassurance in tense situations.

Practicing asanas is a way of learning to exercise self-control. Yoga begins this process by first teaching control of the body, then control of the breath. Through this you learn concentration—control of your thought patterns—and this in turn helps to bring about emotional control. In the long term, yoga has a leveling effect on your whole emotional life. People who practice yoga do not cease to feel, but they become less negatively affected by life's disappointments, less anxiety-ridden, and less dependent for happiness on outside factors such as wealth, success, popularity, and luck. The perpetual need for excitement, gratification, and thrills is replaced by inner peace and contentment.

Reaching this stage of emotional development is to achieve pratyahara or release from the dominance of the senses—the fifth stage on the path of yoga as described by the sage Patañjali (see page 17). Achieving the state of pratyahara signifies that you are ready for the serious practice of dhyana or meditation, through which you may achieve the state of samadhi or oneness with the universal consciousness or spirit. This is the aim of every branch and school of yoga.

A FIRST PRACTICE

This first chapter illustrates and describes ten poses which, carried out in the order shown, make a good introduction to yoga. Together, these ten poses form a complete practice taking perhaps 20 minutes to half an hour—please read the caution note on page 9 before beginning. Working through this program two or three times a week, carrying out the steps in the order given, and concentrating on the accurate positioning of the feet, the arms, and various other parts of the body, will strengthen your muscles, make your joints more flexible, and give you confidence. Like every yoga practice, this one ends with a welcome five to ten minutes of complete relaxation in the corpse pose.

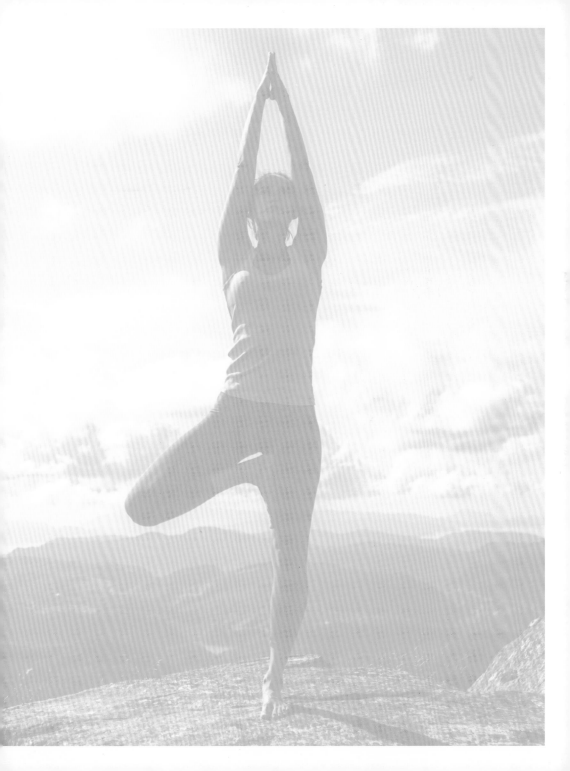

Beginning Yoga

The following pages introduce ten basic yoga poses. They start with sitting and lying down, and go on to analyze standing in tadasana—the mountain pose. Learning to stand properly improves posture, and this can eliminate the often debilitating aches and pains caused by slumping. The standing poses that follow tadasana stretch the legs and spine and, in time, strengthen the whole body.

Step-by-step

These first ten poses, carried out in the given sequence, make a good first class for beginners. Work through each one step-by-step. The instructions in the captions help you achieve the pose without strain, so follow them as closely as you can, holding the stretch at the end for as long as is comfortable.

Triangle, extended side angle, and tree (see pages 46–53 and 58–61) are carried out first on one side of the body, then on the other side. For example, in triangle you bend first to the right, then to the left. And in cross-legged sitting on page 38 you cross the right shin over the left, then the left shin over the right.

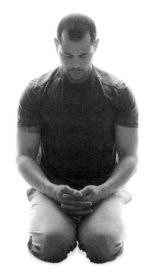

Resting between poses
After an intense stretch, rest briefly in a different position. You might do a standing or a kneeling forward bend, or stand in tadasana for a few seconds.

Do not rush through the poses. Make each movement deliberately, working at your own speed. If you find it hard to stretch into the full pose, do not try to force your body into the unaccustomed position. Joints and muscles that have long been inactive may well feel stiff at first, but if any movement or body position is painful, stop immediately. The rule is: always work to your own potential; stretch as far as you can comfortably, then rest. Next time, you may be able to stretch a little further.

Finishing a pose

To leave a pose, move through the steps in reverse order until you return to the start position. The sequence of poses in this chapter ends with a few minutes of total relaxation in the corpse pose or savasana. This resting pose should make an enjoyable end to every future practice.

Tips on Breathing

Breathe normally while performing all yoga poses, and remember:

- Do not hold your breath while concentrating on the movements.

- Breathe in before a stretch or other exertion and execute the movement on the out-breath.

- Always breathe through the nose unless you have hay fever, a cold, or other sinus problem.

- When relaxing in the corpse pose at the end of the practice, concentrate on quieting the breath, focusing on its rhythm.

SITTING & LYING POSES

The simple cross-legged sitting pose, **sukhasana**, shown on these pages is the basis for many sitting postures. Practiced regularly, it strengthens the back and makes the hips more flexible. The name of the pose at right, **supta tadasana**, or "the lying-down mountain pose" sounds like a contradiction, but this is the basic standing posture performed lying on the mat. It gives a good stretch and relaxes the lower back.

Cross-legged sitting

1 *Sit upright, hands beside your hips, legs stretched out in front, toes turned up. Press your legs and hands down, lift your spine, and bend your left leg and then your right leg, crossing the right shin across the left.*

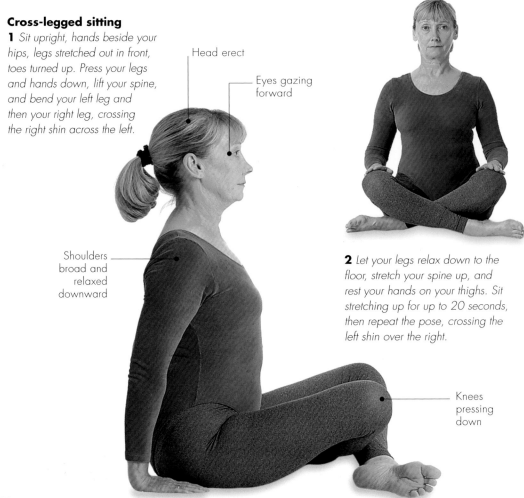

Head erect

Eyes gazing forward

Shoulders broad and relaxed downward

2 *Let your legs relax down to the floor, stretch your spine up, and rest your hands on your thighs. Sit stretching up for up to 20 seconds, then repeat the pose, crossing the left shin over the right.*

Knees pressing down

Lying-down stretch

1 *Lie with the your legs straight, the soles of your feet against a wall, and your arms, palms down, by your sides.*

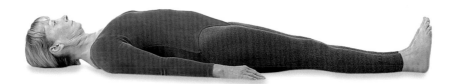

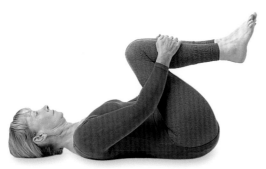

2 *Bend your legs, and adjust the position of your pelvis by bending your knees and raising them to your chest. Then straighten your legs until your heels touch the floor and the soles of your feet press against the wall.*

3 *Lift your arms up and back over your head until the backs of your hands touch the floor behind. Pressing your legs down, stretch from your groins to your fingertips, and from your lower back to your feet. Stretch for up to 20 seconds, then relax.*

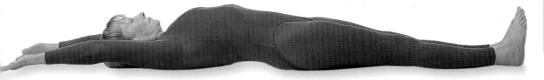

Introducing Floor Poses

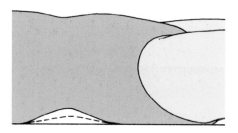

Aligning the spine

If your lower back arches when you lie down, exercising may strain it. To reduce the curve, raise your knees to your chest, then straighten your legs.

Aligning the knees

Sitting on a foam block or a blanket folded two or three times also raises the level of your pelvis, which helps you align your knees. When you cross your legs, your knees need to be the same distance as your hip bones from the mat, but this can be hard to achieve at first. Sitting on a raised level makes it easier to lower the knees. If your knees are stiff, support them on a folded blanket.

The Buddha is often depicted sitting meditating in the lotus pose—each foot placed on the opposite thigh. However, the lotus position is one of many sitting poses and, like the simple cross-legged sitting position on page 38, the alternatives are easier for most people to perform. In this, as in all sitting poses, the lower spine needs to be straight and stretching up. If at first you find it hard to lift your lower back, sit on a blanket folded three or four times, or on a foam block. This supports your back muscles while you work on strengthening them.

Lying-down stretch analyzed

Just lying on the floor seems too simple to need analysis, but attention to the details shown below is the secret of a satisfying stretch.

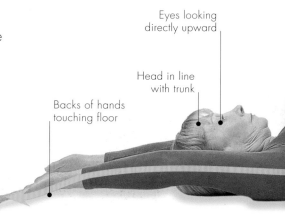

Eyes looking directly upward

Head in line with trunk

Backs of hands touching floor

Lying-down poses

Many yoga poses are performed lying on the mat. Supta tadasana, the lying-down stretch on page 39, is a wonderful whole-body stretch. Press the sitting bones (see pages 26–27) toward your feet, and your legs and heels down, and stretch from your hips to your head, along your arms to your fingertips, and along your legs, pressing your feet into the wall.

Points to Watch

- When you stretch toward your hands while sitting or lying, keep your rib cage in its natural alignment so that the lower ribs do not protrude.

- Keep your sitting bones stretching down to the floor in the sitting pose and toward your feet in the lying-down stretch, while lifting your hip bones toward your head.

- While stretching your spine up, keep your shoulders broad but relaxed downward so your shoulder blades remain flat against your ribs.

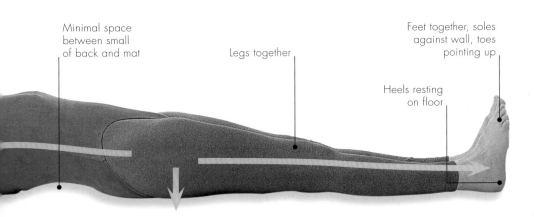

Minimal space between small of back and mat

Legs together

Feet together, soles against wall, toes pointing up

Heels resting on floor

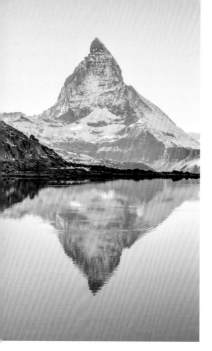

Mountain pose

The basic standing pose in yoga is called tadasana or mountain pose because you stand as upright and immobile as a mountain.

STANDING Tadasana, the standing mountain
pose, can be practiced indoors or out, waiting for a train, for instance, or standing in a line. It is the basis of good posture and consequently of good health. Making a habit of standing in tadasana corrects poor posture and can make back and joint pains disappear so that your whole body feels healthier and lighter. It also deepens your understanding of every other yoga pose.

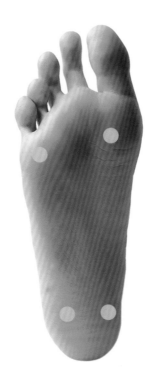

Balancing points

Spread each foot, broadening and lengthening it, stretching the toes forward, and balancing the weight of your body evenly on each of the four key balancing points on the sole of the foot, shown in this diagram.

Keeping your ribs in their normal position, lift your breastbone and stretch across your upper chest and shoulders. Move your shoulders back and down, flattening the shoulder blades

Straighten your neck to align your head with your spine and position your chin parallel to the floor, and direct your gaze forward. Hold the position for 20 seconds, breathing gently

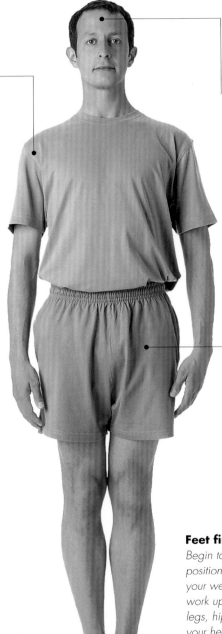

Stretch your legs up, lift your trunk from your hips, and stretch your sitting bones downward. Tighten your thigh muscles to press your thighs back

Feet first

Begin tadasana by thinking about the positioning of your feet and the fall of your weight down to the floor. Then work up your body, positioning your legs, hips, trunk, shoulders, and, finally, your head. As you hold the position, you should be standing as erect and steady as a mountain.

Stand with your feet together, distributing your weight evenly on the balls and heels of both feet, big toes, heels, ankles, and knees touching, arms relaxed by your sides

Improving Posture

An erect spine is the basis of good posture, but this does not mean that the spine should be ramrod-straight. A spine that is correctly aligned lifts from the sacrum—the shield-shaped bone at its base which forms the back of the pelvis—and stretches up, falling into its three natural curves (shown on pages 26–27).

Aligning the pelvis

Clearly, the key to this upright posture is the correct positioning of the pelvis. To lift your spine from the sacrum, your pelvis must be properly aligned, so the best way to start all yoga poses is by checking and adjusting it. Do this in the mountain pose on pages 42–43 by stretching your sitting bones toward the floor, and lifting the front of your body from the hip bones.

If your back muscles are weak, the pelvis tends to tilt forward and you lift from the waist instead of from the hips. In time, simply practicing the mountain pose—tadasana—will correct this defect by strengthening the spine's supporting muscles. This will enable you to lift from the hips without support in standing and sitting poses.

Achieving stability

Beginning the pose by distributing your body weight equally between the key points on the heel and forefoot (see page 42) gives you stability. Lift the arches of your feet without disturbing your balance and maintain your stability as you stretch your legs up, lift your trunk from the pelvis, raise your breastbone, and align your lower back. Make this pose part of your daily routine and any back pain you experience will soon disappear.

Points to Watch

- Straighten your legs without locking your knees by lifting the kneecaps and stretching the leg muscles up.

- Keep your hips back, in line with your ankle bones.

- Do not pull your abdomen in. Lift the front of your pelvis and your abdomen will move back toward your spine.

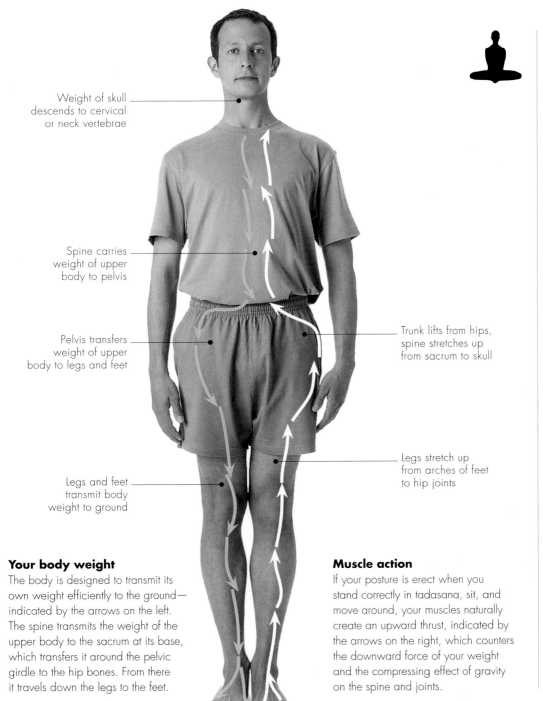

Weight of skull descends to cervical or neck vertebrae

Spine carries weight of upper body to pelvis

Pelvis transfers weight of upper body to legs and feet

Legs and feet transmit body weight to ground

Trunk lifts from hips, spine stretches up from sacrum to skull

Legs stretch up from arches of feet to hip joints

Your body weight

The body is designed to transmit its own weight efficiently to the ground—indicated by the arrows on the left. The spine transmits the weight of the upper body to the sacrum at its base, which transfers it around the pelvic girdle to the hip bones. From there it travels down the legs to the feet.

Muscle action

If your posture is erect when you stand correctly in tadasana, sit, and move around, your muscles naturally create an upward thrust, indicated by the arrows on the right, which counters the downward force of your weight and the compressing effect of gravity on the spine and joints.

TRIANGLE

Utthita trikonasana—the triangle pose—starts you working on improving the flexibility of your hips and legs. Like all the standing poses, you begin in the mountain pose and go on to make a series of triangle shapes with your body, legs, and arms.

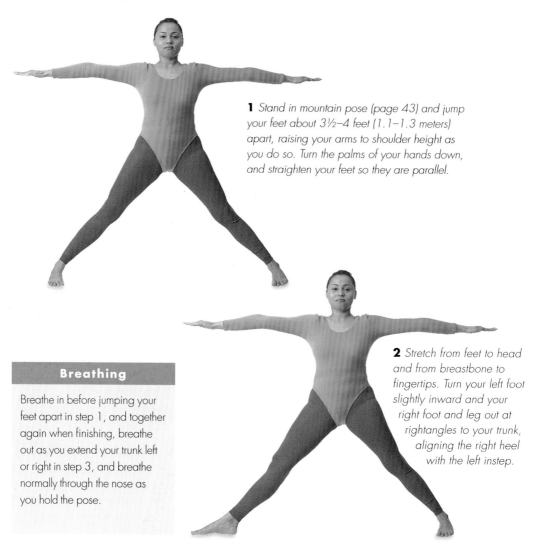

1 *Stand in mountain pose (page 43) and jump your feet about 3½–4 feet (1.1–1.3 meters) apart, raising your arms to shoulder height as you do so. Turn the palms of your hands down, and straighten your feet so they are parallel.*

2 *Stretch from feet to head and from breastbone to fingertips. Turn your left foot slightly inward and your right foot and leg out at rightangles to your trunk, aligning the right heel with the left instep.*

Breathing

Breathe in before jumping your feet apart in step 1, and together again when finishing, breathe out as you extend your trunk left or right in step 3, and breathe normally through the nose as you hold the pose.

3 *Breathe in and stretch up, then breathe out and bend from the hips to the right until your right hand touches the floor beside and slightly behind your right calf. Align your trunk with your legs, stretch your left arm up in line with your right arm, and turn your head to look up at your left hand. Hold, breathing normally, for 10–15 seconds.*

Using a Wall

Practicing the pose with your back against a wall—represented by the tinted frame of this box—makes it easier to keep your shoulders back, in line with your hips and leg, and your legs and trunk ligned.

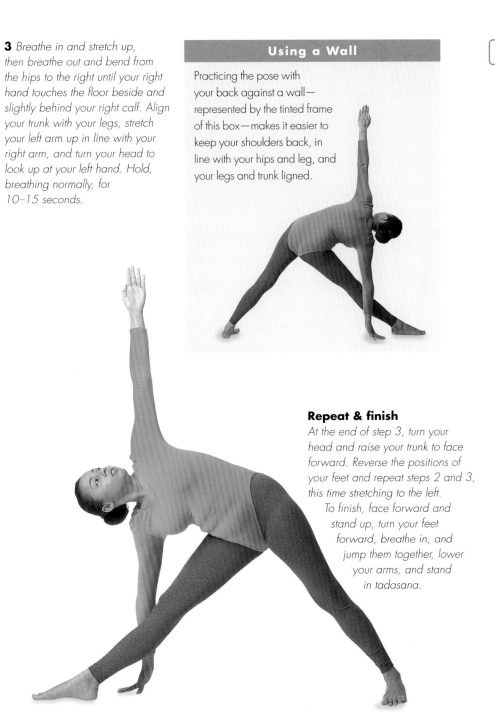

Repeat & finish

At the end of step 3, turn your head and raise your trunk to face forward. Reverse the positions of your feet and repeat steps 2 and 3, this time stretching to the left.
To finish, face forward and stand up, turn your feet forward, breathe in, and jump them together, lower your arms, and stand in tadasana.

Focus on Alignment

Good alignment of all the body parts is the key to triangle pose, and that alignment depends on whole-body stretching. The pose begins with a stretch: a good tadasana (see pages 42–45) lifting all the way up from the arches of the feet to the crown of the head. Then after you jump your legs astride, pause, feet parallel, to stretch your legs, lift your breastbone, and extend your arms out to the fingertips while keeping your shoulders back and down.

Extending the stretch

Before bending from the hips it is important to continue the stretch, lifting up from the groins and opening the chest. Keep your legs stretching up, your sitting bones (see pages 26–27) extending down toward the floor, and lift along both sides of the trunk, and you can be confident you are achieving the pose even if you are unable to reach the floor with your hand. Rest the hand on your leg, a chair seat, or foam yoga blocks instead, and concentrate on stretching while keeping your legs and back aligned. The stiffness in your hips will

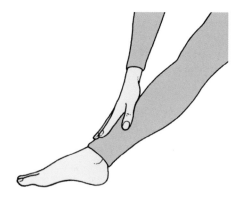

Achieving the pose
If when bending from the hips in step 3 you can reach only your calf at first, rest your hand on your leg, then work lower until you can reach the floor.

Points to Watch

- Do not allow the side of the trunk that is uppermost to roll forward. Revolve it back as if pressing it against a wall.

- Keep your thighs pressing back.

- Turn your right leg out to the right and keep your left shin facing forward.

soon ease, enabling you to lower your hand a little more each time you practice the triangle pose.

Triangle pose analyzed

Once you have learned the basic steps for the triangle pose on pages 46–47, you need to work on the details. It is easy to allow the trunk to roll forward or the legs to turn in. The details make all the difference in every yoga pose, so concentrating on the points in the diagram below and stretching in the direction shown by the arrows will help you improve and benefit.

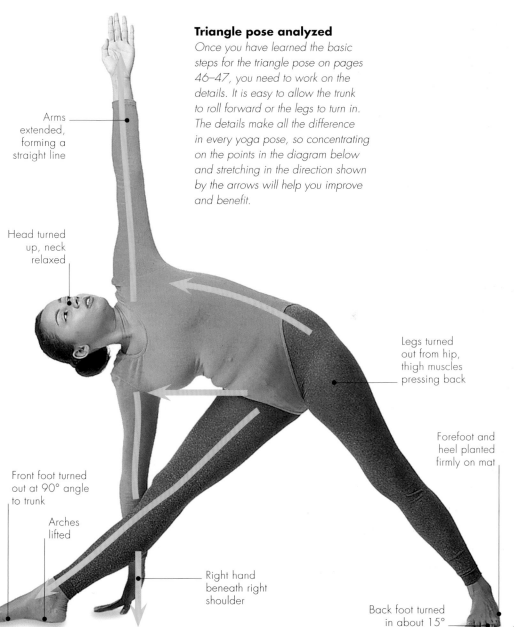

Arms extended, forming a straight line

Head turned up, neck relaxed

Legs turned out from hip, thigh muscles pressing back

Forefoot and heel planted firmly on mat

Front foot turned out at 90° angle to trunk

Arches lifted

Right hand beneath right shoulder

Back foot turned in about 15°

49

EXTENDED SIDE ANGLE

Triangles continue to be the theme of **utthita parsvakonasana**, illustrated here, in which you stretch from your feet, along your sides to your fingertips, forming a triangle with your whole body. This pose tones and aligns ankles, calves, knees, and thighs, and it is said to slim the waist and hips.

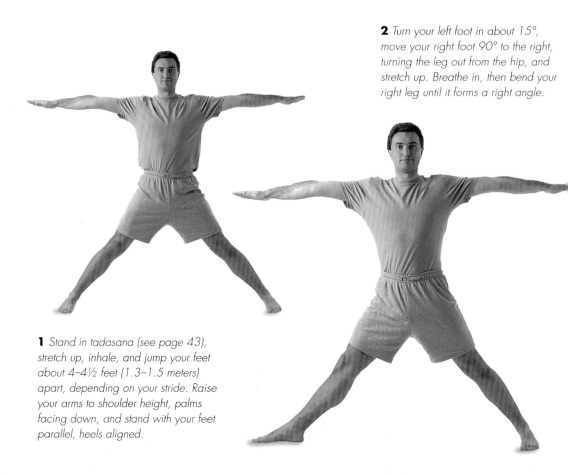

2 *Turn your left foot in about 15°, move your right foot 90° to the right, turning the leg out from the hip, and stretch up. Breathe in, then bend your right leg until it forms a right angle.*

1 *Stand in tadasana (see page 43), stretch up, inhale, and jump your feet about 4–4½ feet (1.3–1.5 meters) apart, depending on your stride. Raise your arms to shoulder height, palms facing down, and stand with your feet parallel, heels aligned.*

Your Stride

Several standing poses require you to jump your feet between 3 and 4½ feet (1–1.5 meters) apart, but how far you can jump your feet apart depends on your leg length—3–3½ feet (1–1.1 meters) may be right for a short person, 4–4½ feet (1.3–1.5 meters) for a long-legged person.

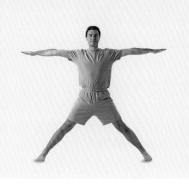

3 *Keeping your trunk facing forward and your arms extended out at shoulder level, stretch up, bend your trunk to the right, and place your right hand beside your right ankle. Your left arm extends vertically upward.*

4 *Rotate your left arm to the right and move it toward your head until the arm almost touches your ear and the left side of your body forms a straight line from foot to fingers. Look up, and hold for up to 10–15 seconds.*

Repeat & finish

Turn to face forward, raise your trunk, straighten your right leg, and turn your feet to the front. Repeat steps 2 and 3, bending to the left, and stretching your right arm up.

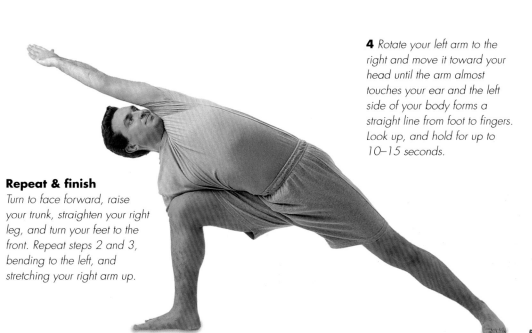

Side-stretches

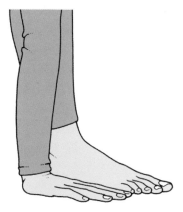

Working on the pose
When you bend your knee in step 2, your shin must make a 90° angle to the floor. As you bend to the side in step 3, place your right hand beside your right ankle, in line with the foot.

The extended side-angle pose shown on pages 50–51 gives both sides of the body a stretch, and to benefit fully you should maintain the stretch from step 1, when you inhale and stretch up from the groins and out all the way from your breastbone to your fingertips.

Think carefully about the position of your feet when you turn them in step 2. Move the toes of your left foot in slightly, pressing the outside of the foot into the floor and lifting the arch, stretching the

left leg up and turning it out from the hip to face forward. Press your thigh muscles back, then rotate your right leg out from the hip joint, turning the right foot at right angles to the trunk, and aligning it with the left instep.

Bending to the side

Maintain the upward stretch and keep both your legs turned out at the hip as you bend from the hips to the right. Keep your trunk facing forward as you extend your right side along your right thigh, and place your right hand beside the ankle directly beneath your right shoulder. If you find it difficult to reach the floor, rest your elbow on your thigh, or your right hand on a foam yoga block placed on the floor beside your right foot. Then, as you gradually begin to straighten your left arm, turn it to the right and stretch it up and to the right. At this point in the exercise the left side of your body will form a straight line from the outer edge of the left foot, along the line of the straightened left leg, to the hip, up the left side of the trunk, and along the left arm.

Points to Watch

- Keep your head, shoulders, trunk, and hips in line. Do not let your shoulders and trunk roll forward.

- As you turn your feet, rotate your leg in the same direction from the hip joint. Feet, leg, and knee should all face the same way.

Extended side angle analyzed

Work on the details to improve in step 4 of extended side-angle pose on page 51.

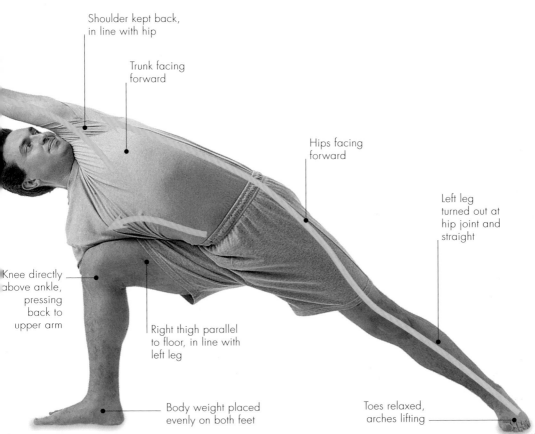

Shoulder kept back, in line with hip

Trunk facing forward

Hips facing forward

Left leg turned out at hip joint and straight

Knee directly above ankle, pressing back to upper arm

Right thigh parallel to floor, in line with left leg

Body weight placed evenly on both feet

Toes relaxed, arches lifting

FORWARD BENDS

Something relaxing is needed after the exertion of the last two poses, and these forward bends are particularly good for resting the back. They are the first of several classic forward bends in this book, some performed while sitting, others while standing. All can be very restful.

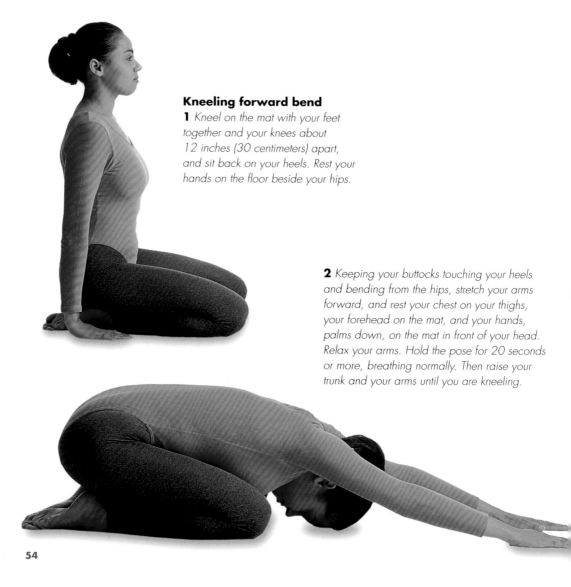

Kneeling forward bend

1 *Kneel on the mat with your feet together and your knees about 12 inches (30 centimeters) apart, and sit back on your heels. Rest your hands on the floor beside your hips.*

2 *Keeping your buttocks touching your heels and bending from the hips, stretch your arms forward, and rest your chest on your thighs, your forehead on the mat, and your hands, palms down, on the mat in front of your head. Relax your arms. Hold the pose for 20 seconds or more, breathing normally. Then raise your trunk and your arms until you are kneeling.*

Standing forward bend

1 *Stand about 3 feet (1 meter) from a chair back, your feet 12 inches (30 centimeters) apart, your weight evenly balanced on the balls and heels of both feet. Stretch your legs up, inhale, and raise your arms above your head, lifting from hips to fingertips.*

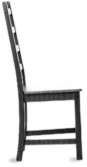

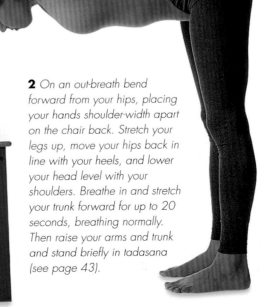

2 *On an out-breath bend forward from your hips, placing your hands shoulder-width apart on the chair back. Stretch your legs up, move your hips back in line with your heels, and lower your head level with your shoulders. Breathe in and stretch your trunk forward for up to 20 seconds, breathing normally. Then raise your arms and trunk and stand briefly in tadasana (see page 43).*

Introducing Forward Bends

Forward bends calm the mind and rest the body. They position the head level with or lower than the trunk, and this is said to refresh the nerves. They counter the compressing effects of gravity on the spine by stretching it, separating the vertebrae. A kneeling forward bend can be an antidote to backaches caused by spending most of the day on your feet.

If at first it is difficult to kneel, rest your knees on a folded blanket. You can perform this pose with knees and feet together, but bending forward with your knees apart makes it easier to keep your heels touching your buttocks and your forehead on the mat. If you do not achieve this at first, rest your head on a blanket folded two or three times, or a foam block, and, if necessary, place one on your heels to sit back onto. Stiffness in your knees, hips, and spine will soon ease, allowing you to dispense with these aids.

Kneeling forward bend analyzed

Once you have learned the basic steps for the kneeling forward bend on page 54, work on improving these details.

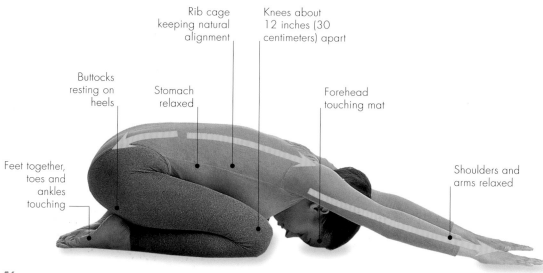

Rib cage keeping natural alignment

Knees about 12 inches (30 centimeters) apart

Buttocks resting on heels

Stomach relaxed

Forehead touching mat

Feet together, toes and ankles touching

Shoulders and arms relaxed

Bending from the hips

The standing forward bend on page 55 will loosen the muscles and tendons at the back of your thighs, but because you bend only to hip level you will not stretch them too far, too quickly. It is essential to bend from the hips, so choose a chair (or a stool or a table) that reaches roughly to hip level. If it is higher, the tendons will not be well stretched, and if it is too low for your height, you will tend to bend from the waist. Straighten your legs only as far as you can without feeling pain.

Standing forward bend analyzed

Working on the points shown below will help you improve the standing forward bend on page 55.

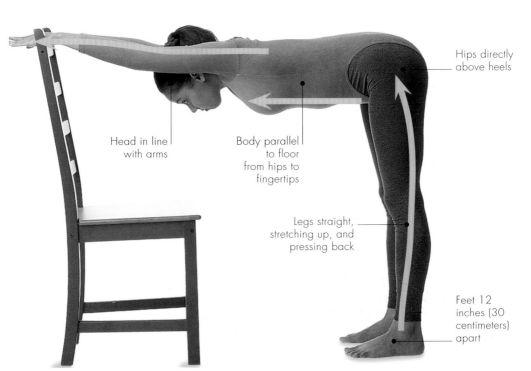

Head in line with arms

Body parallel to floor from hips to fingertips

Legs straight, stretching up, and pressing back

Hips directly above heels

Feet 12 inches (30 centimeters) apart

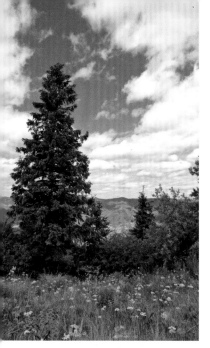

Inspiration from nature
In tree pose your joined hands stretch skyward like the topmost branches of a mountain pine.

TREE Striving to achieve perfect balance is fundamental to all aspects of yoga. You may wobble when you first try **vrksasana**, the tree pose, but with perseverance you quickly find your ankles and legs strengthen and your balance improves. Having greater confidence in your balance gives you more poise. The tree pose also stretches your body from your toes to your head and arms, toning the muscles of your legs, lifting your spine, and straightening your back.

1 *Stand in tadasana (see page 43) stretching up. Move your weight to your left leg, turn your right leg out at the hip, and bend the knee, grasping the ankle with your right hand.*

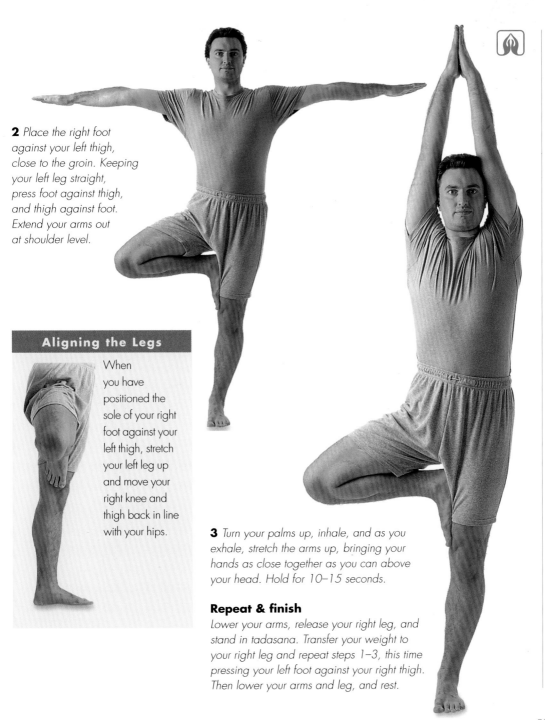

2 *Place the right foot against your left thigh, close to the groin. Keeping your left leg straight, press foot against thigh, and thigh against foot. Extend your arms out at shoulder level.*

Aligning the Legs

When you have positioned the sole of your right foot against your left thigh, stretch your left leg up and move your right knee and thigh back in line with your hips.

3 *Turn your palms up, inhale, and as you exhale, stretch the arms up, bringing your hands as close together as you can above your head. Hold for 10–15 seconds.*

Repeat & finish

Lower your arms, release your right leg, and stand in tadasana. Transfer your weight to your right leg and repeat steps 1–3, this time pressing your left foot against your right thigh. Then lower your arms and leg, and rest.

59

Improving Balance

Balancing in the tree pose on pages 58–59 depends on beginning by stretching up in a good tadasana. As you transfer your weight to the leg you are going to stand on, stretch that leg up still more strongly. Your hip joints may be stiff at first, making it hard to raise the foot to the top of the opposite thigh, but you can raise your foot and keep it lifted with a belt around the ankle. In time the joints ease. Although the belt prevents you from raising both arms, it enables you to stand upright while stretching.

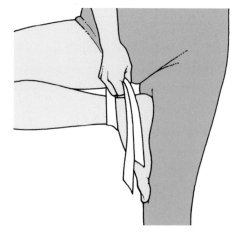

Working on the pose
If you have trouble keeping the foot in position against the thigh, or if your arms are short and you cannot reach your ankle, wind a belt around the ankle and hold the belt in the same hand.

The key to balance

Keeping the raised foot pressing into the thigh of the standing leg, close to the groin, and the thigh pressing into the heel and sole of the foot is the key to balancing in this posture. Imagine your foot and the inside of your thigh acting like a magnet, pressing into each other. Extending your sitting bones toward the mat and focusing your gaze on some object at eye level also makes it easier to maintain your balance.

Making the most of the stretch

Once you feel balanced, slowly raise both arms until they are level with your shoulders, palms facing down. (If one hand is holding a belt, place your free hand on your hip.) Keeping your head up, rotate your arms to turn your palms up. On an out-breath, raise your arms above your head. Breathe normally as you hold the pose, and really stretch up from your feet to your fingertips. Enjoy the stretch.

Points to Watch

- Keep the thigh and knee of your bent leg back in line with your trunk.
- Keep your hips level and aligned.
- Keep your sitting bones stretching downward.
- As you stretch your arms up, lift your breastbone, but do not push your rib cage forward.

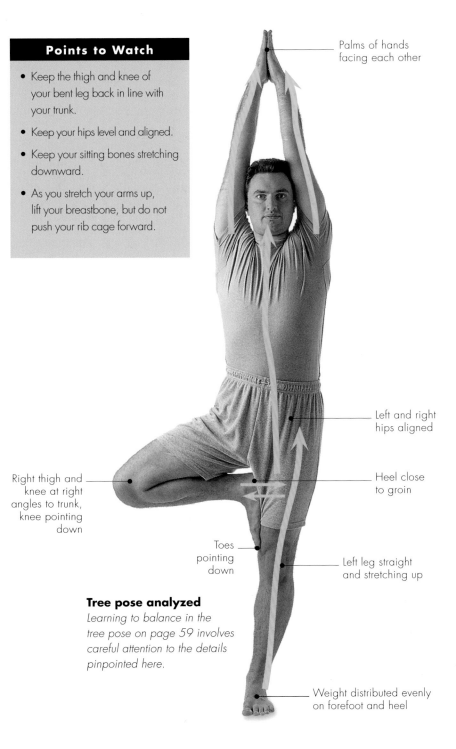

Palms of hands facing each other

Left and right hips aligned

Right thigh and knee at right angles to trunk, knee pointing down

Heel close to groin

Toes pointing down

Left leg straight and stretching up

Tree pose analyzed

Learning to balance in the tree pose on page 59 involves careful attention to the details pinpointed here.

Weight distributed evenly on forefoot and heel

LEG-STRETCH

LEG-STRETCH **Urdhva prasarita padasana** is a wonderful pick-me-up if you feel fatigued or if your feet or legs ache, and a restful posture to insert briefly between some of the more complex poses in Chapter 4. Some authorities recommend it for relief of gas. Do it without the support of a wall if you want to tighten your stomach muscles and slim your abdomen.

1 *Lie on one side with legs bent and both buttocks touching a wall.*

2 *Keeping your buttocks against the wall, roll onto your back, and stretch both legs together up the wall so your thighs, calves, and heels press against it.*

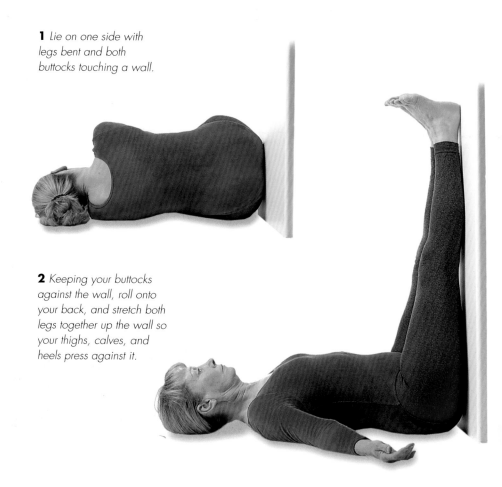

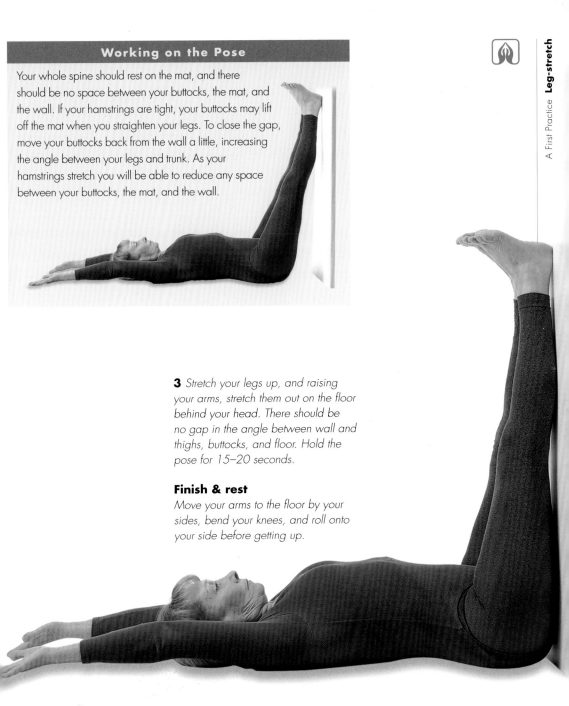

Working on the Pose

Your whole spine should rest on the mat, and there should be no space between your buttocks, the mat, and the wall. If your hamstrings are tight, your buttocks may lift off the mat when you straighten your legs. To close the gap, move your buttocks back from the wall a little, increasing the angle between your legs and trunk. As your hamstrings stretch you will be able to reduce any space between your buttocks, the mat, and the wall.

3 *Stretch your legs up, and raising your arms, stretch them out on the floor behind your head. There should be no gap in the angle between wall and thighs, buttocks, and floor. Hold the pose for 15–20 seconds.*

Finish & rest
Move your arms to the floor by your sides, bend your knees, and roll onto your side before getting up.

63

Ending with Relaxation

The most relaxing pose of all is the corpse pose, **savasana I**. It relaxes your muscles after stretching and rests your mind, which has been concentrating on movement. You begin by stretching your back, your legs and feet, and your arms and hands, then close your eyes and focus your mind on each part of the body in turn—relax the muscles in each limb, and in the joints, release any tension in your stomach muscles and your spine, soften your jaw, and eradicate any tension in the muscles of your face and around your eyes. Focusing on each part of the body in turn and on slow, rhythmic breathing helps keep your mind free of encroaching thoughts that may make you tense up.

Antidote to stress

Your first practice should end with a few minutes of complete relaxation of mind and body in savasana I. This completes the practice, preparing you physically and mentally to rejoin your everyday life. These poses can be a useful antidote to stress and tension outside practice time. Spending five to ten minutes alone in savasana clears the mind and makes difficult situations easier to handle.

Corpse pose analyzed

Follow the steps for savasana I opposite, check these details, then focus your mind on your breathing and on relaxing each part of your body.

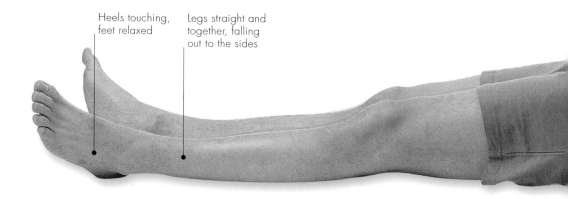

Heels touching, feet relaxed

Legs straight and together, falling out to the sides

1 *Sit with your legs together, knees bent, and hands on the floor beside your hips. Lie back, gently lowering your spine until your head touches the mat. Stretching your sitting bones toward your feet, slowly straighten your legs and draw them together until your feet touch.*

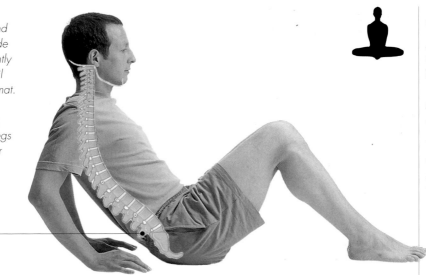

Spine uncurling, vertebra by vertebra

2 *Lift your head to check your legs and body are aligned, then lower it in line with your trunk. Draw your legs together so your feet touch, and stretch your legs, pushing your heels away from your head and your toes toward it, then let your legs fall apart. Rotate your arms from the shoulders until your palms face up. Stretch from shoulders to fingertips, then relax them, close your eyes, and slowly relax your whole body.*

Palms turned up

Arms resting a short distance from the sides

Head in line with body

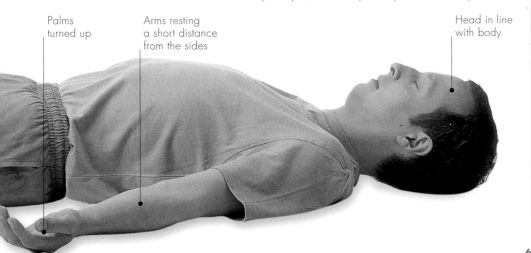

CLASSIC POSES

When you feel familiar with the ten basic poses in Chapter 3, you may wish to learn some new ones. This chapter illustrates and gives you step-by-step instructions showing how to perform some 40 classic poses. The six major categories: standing poses, sitting poses, floor poses, sitting twists, backbends, and inverted poses, follow on from each other, and the chapter ends with a few fun exercises for the shoulders and hands.

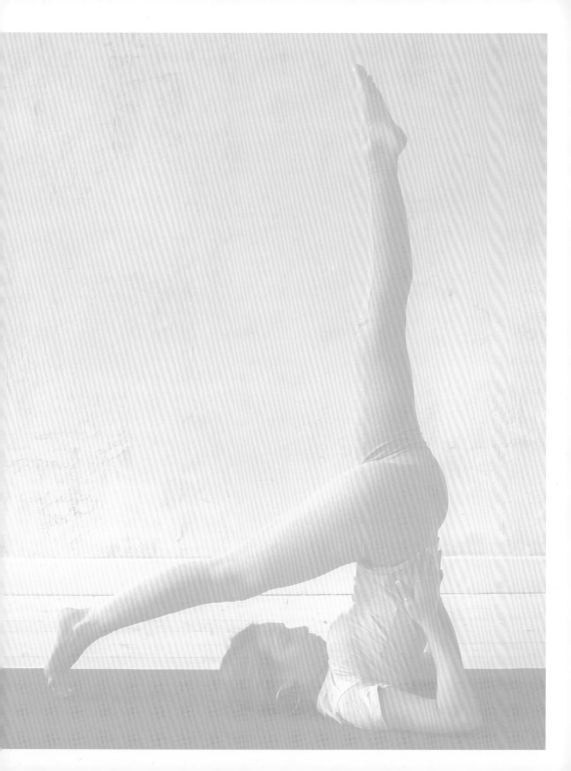

Making Progress

The ten poses in Chapter 3 are the foundation of many asanas. As you progress, you learn new ones, yet you never stop practicing those you learned first. People who have studied yoga for years continue to work on improving tadasana. Every pose is a lifelong learning experience.

Standing poses

You need not work through every pose in this chapter in the order given, but beginners should start with some of the standing postures on pages 70–105 because they build stamina and improve flexibility. Practicing the less demanding standing poses (indicated by a light blue icon in the top right-hand corner of the page), with a wall behind you for support, will help you regain strength after illness. But it is unwise to work on holding stretches for longer and longer periods. The best approach is to hold a pose for five to ten seconds, then rest and repeat it. You are sure to see a steady improvement.

Holistic practice

All yoga poses work on the whole body, so if, for example, your shoulders feel tense, you should not spend all your practice time repeating shoulder exercises. Standing, sitting, and floor poses will also help loosen them.

The more vigorous sitting and floor postures that follow the standing poses may need more effort at first. But do not

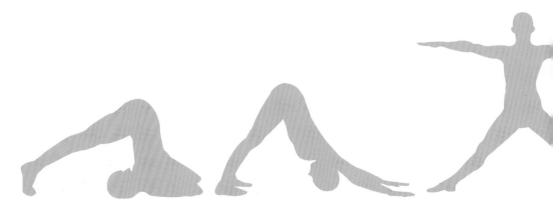

try so hard that you strain your body. Give it time to gain flexibility and strength, and be satisfied to achieve your personal best. There are no goals to score in yoga. Work at stretching and gradual extension, and if a pose seems to stress any part of your body, stop, and work on less demanding postures until your flexibility improves.

Support & protection

Learn each pose by following the steps shown in the color photographs. The black-and-white pages that follow analyze the pose. They help you achieve it by using foam yoga blocks or folded blankets to support your back or rest your weight, and belts to help you stretch.

Always use folded blankets or foam blocks for support during the inverted poses on pages 186–93. And when getting to your feet from a lying position after any floor pose, roll onto one side before getting up, to protect your back from strain. Keep these warnings in mind, but do not limit yourself to a narrow range of poses. Be adventurous and you may be surprised at how much you can achieve.

Exploring the poses

Be willing to try out a new pose, however difficult it seems. Some poses will seem astonishingly simple, and you will need to work to achieve others.

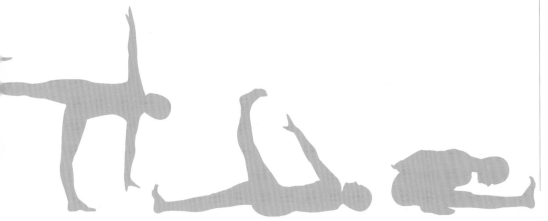

EXTENDED LEG-STRETCHES
These two poses work on extending the limbs to their fullest extent in order to improve the balance and strengthen the legs. They are assisted versions of the pose for beginners, for which you need a piece of solid furniture or perhaps a ledge the right height for you to rest your heel on with your leg straightened.

Utthita hasta padangusthasana I
1 *Stand in tadasana (see page 43), about 3 feet (1 meter) from the chair or ledge, stretch your legs and spine up, then bend your right leg and place your right heel on the chair or ledge.*

2 *Wind a belt around your right foot, and holding it with both hands, stand upright, arms straight. Stretch your left leg up, and stretch your right leg by pressing your foot against the belt. Hold the pose for about 20 seconds.*

Repeat & finish
Remove the belt and lower your right foot to the floor. Stretch up for a few seconds, then repeat steps 1 and 2, this time raising your left leg.

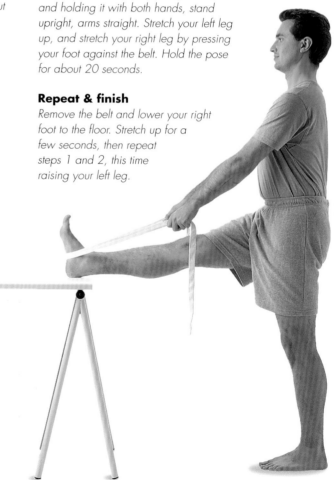

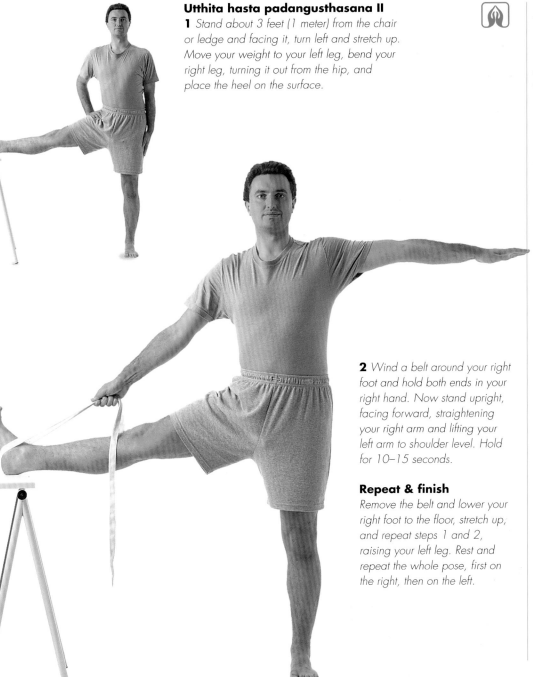

Utthita hasta padangusthasana II

1 *Stand about 3 feet (1 meter) from the chair or ledge and facing it, turn left and stretch up. Move your weight to your left leg, bend your right leg, turning it out from the hip, and place the heel on the surface.*

2 *Wind a belt around your right foot and hold both ends in your right hand. Now stand upright, facing forward, straightening your right arm and lifting your left arm to shoulder level. Hold for 10–15 seconds.*

Repeat & finish

Remove the belt and lower your right foot to the floor, stretch up, and repeat steps 1 and 2, raising your left leg. Rest and repeat the whole pose, first on the right, then on the left.

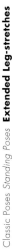

Exercising the Legs

For utthita hasta padangusthasana I and II on pages 70–71 you need to find a heavy piece of furniture or a ledge at the right level to rest your foot— high enough to make you stretch your legs, keeping your hips level, but not so high that you cannot straighten them. Some people can lift their legs quite high, so check first by standing about 3 feet (1 meter) away, steady yourself, lift one foot, and bending at the knee, place your heel on it. Now try to straighten your raised leg. If you cannot, the ledge or chair is too high. As you practice you will find you need to raise the height gradually by placing a foam yoga block (or blocks) on it and resting your foot on top. If you use a chair back, place the chair seat against a wall for stability.

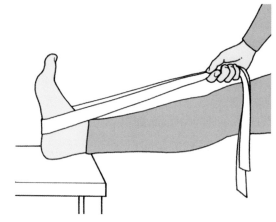

Achieving the pose
Winding a belt around the arch of your raised foot will help you stretch the leg by pressing the foot against the belt with your toes facing up.

Points to Watch

- Keep the leg you are standing on straight and stretching up, foot pointing forward.

- Keep your trunk and hips facing forward, and your hip bones level.

- Stretch your sitting bones down toward the mat and lift up from the groins.

Moving on

You can take these two poses to progressively more advanced levels. As your legs gain flexibility, you will be able to lift your leg high without the help of a chair or a belt. Eventually, you will be able to raise your foot to shoulder height and keep your leg straight while holding the big toe with the hand on the same side of the body. But that can take years to achieve.

Extended leg-stretches analyzed

Although this diagram shows the leg-stretch on page 71—utthita hasta padangusthasana II—these details will also help you keep your balance in utthita hasta padangusthasana I, shown on page 70.

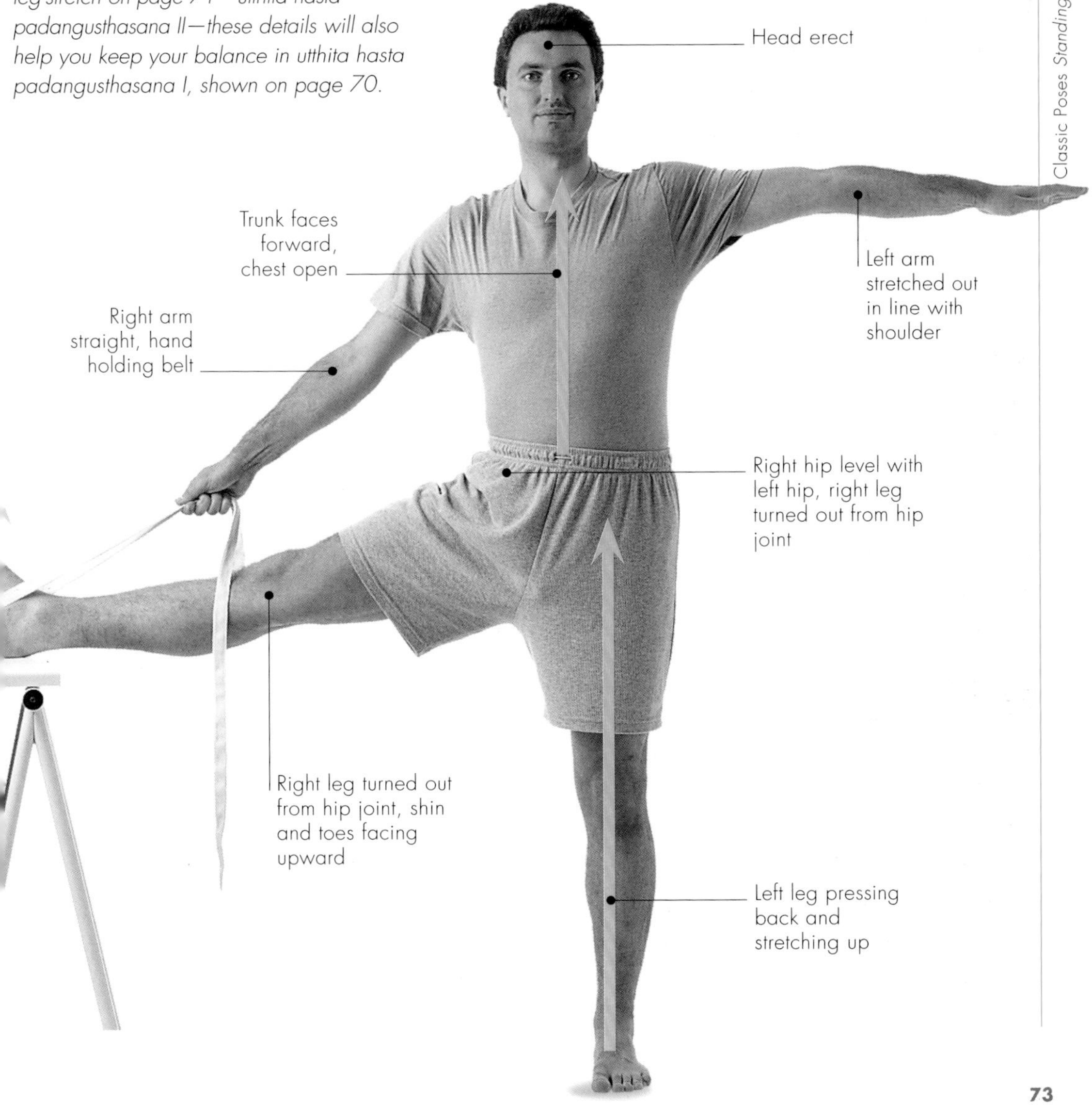

Head erect

Trunk faces forward, chest open

Right arm straight, hand holding belt

Left arm stretched out in line with shoulder

Right hip level with left hip, right leg turned out from hip joint

Right leg turned out from hip joint, shin and toes facing upward

Left leg pressing back and stretching up

EXERCISING THE BACK

The **Marichyasana** and **uttanasana I** poses turn and extend the spine to make it more flexible. The standing pose introduces the twists, which rotate the vertebrae, and the standing forward bend, at right, bends the spine forward from the hips (please read the caution note on page 9 before attempting these poses). Together these poses give the spine an intense and satisfying stretch.

3 *Place your right hand on the wall and press with the fingertips to push your right side away and your left side toward it. Twist for 10–15 seconds.*

Repeat & finish

Lower your hands, turn to face forward, and stand in tadasana, then repeat the pose, turning the chair and twisting to the left side.

Standing chair twist

1 *Stand beside the chair with your right side close to the wall, feet together, hands by your sides. Place your right foot on the chair, and stretch up.*

2 *Put your left hand on your right knee and pull on it to turn your left side toward the wall.*

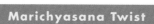

Marichyasana Twist

The pose shown on this page, called Marichyasana because it is based on an exercise devised by a sage, Marichi, exercises the spine by twisting it. Position a chair so its seat touches a wall, and place two foam yoga blocks on the seat and also touching the wall, and place your foot on the blocks.

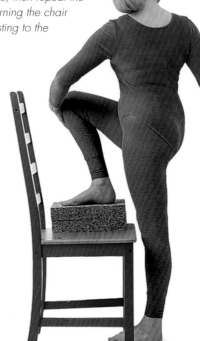

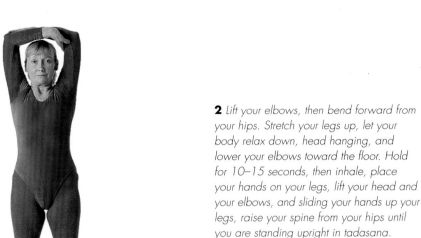

2 *Lift your elbows, then bend forward from your hips. Stretch your legs up, let your body relax down, head hanging, and lower your elbows toward the floor. Hold for 10–15 seconds, then inhale, place your hands on your legs, lift your head and your elbows, and sliding your hands up your legs, raise your spine from your hips until you are standing upright in tadasana.*

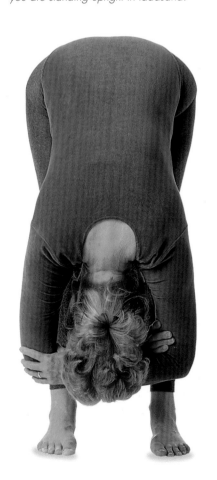

Standing forward bend

1 *Stand with your feet parallel, hip-width apart, your weight evenly balanced. Stretch up from your feet, and lifting from your hips, raise your arms above your head. Bending your elbows, catch hold of the upper arms just above the elbows.*

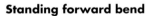

Uttanasana I

When you feel you can do the simplified standing forward bend in Chapter 3 easily, move to uttanasana I, the slightly more advanced version shown here. This pose stretches the whole spine, yet it is perfect for resting between more complex poses.

Achieving a Supple Spine

The secret of twisting is to lift and stretch, so begin the simple twist on page 74 by standing erect, the crown of your head facing the ceiling. Stretch the leg on which you stand strongly up, pressing it firmly back at the same time. Stretch your sitting bones toward the floor and your spine up, and exhale as you turn. Your arm acts as a fulcrum as the hand pressing against the wall levers one side of your body away from the wall, and the hand pulling against your knee draws the other side closer to it. This combined action helps you turn a degree or two further.

Making a forward bend

Stretch your legs strongly upward before bending forward in uttanasana I on page 75, lift from the hip bones, and extend the trunk upward. Stretch your arms as you raise them, and with your hands keeping hold of your upper arms, lift your elbows high, then breathe out as you bend forward—from the hips, not from the waist. This is a relaxing pose, for the body hangs from the hips while the legs do the hard work.

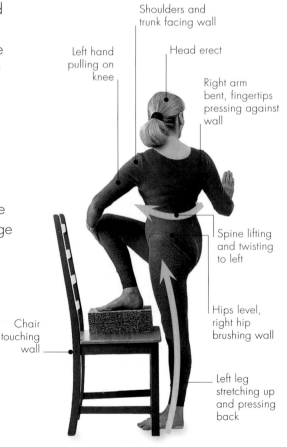

Shoulders and trunk facing wall

Left hand pulling on knee

Head erect

Right arm bent, fingertips pressing against wall

Spine lifting and twisting to left

Hips level, right hip brushing wall

Chair touching wall

Left leg stretching up and pressing back

Standing chair twist
Think about the details shown in the diagram, right, to achieve the Marichyasana twist on page 74.

Trunk bending
from hips, left
and right hips
aligned

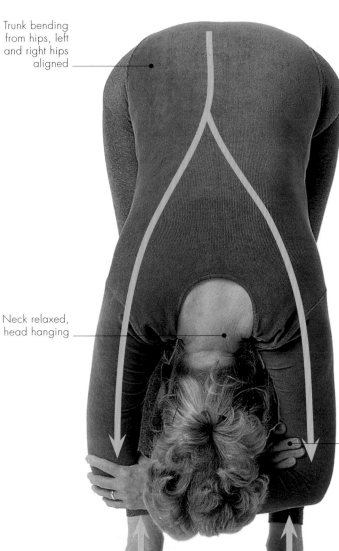

Standing forward bend analyzed

The key to achieving the standing forward bend on page 75 is to think about stretching the legs strongly up, while concentrating on the points shown here. If you have a slipped disk or other back problem, you should not attempt this pose. Instead, continue to practice the version shown on page 55.

Neck relaxed,
head hanging

Opposite hands holding
upper arms, elbows
relaxed downward

Feet apart, weight
evenly distributed

WARRIOR II

Virabhadrasana is the name of a great warrior in an epic poem by the 5th-century Indian dramatist, Kalidasa. There are several warrior poses. **Virabhadrasana II**, the first and simplest, develops the muscles of the calves and thighs and is a good preparation for the more advanced standing poses, especially the forward bends.

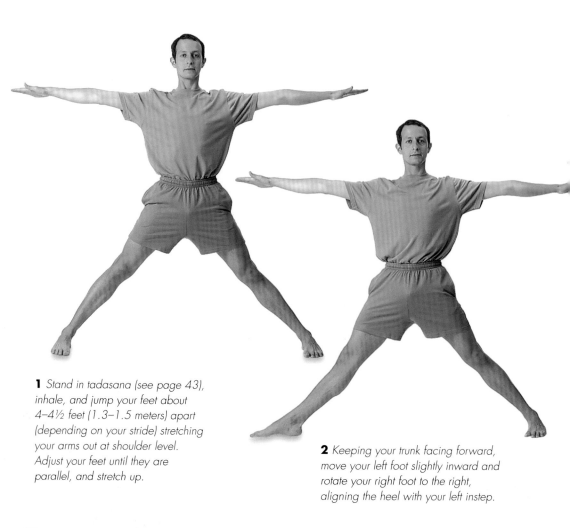

1 Stand in tadasana (see page 43), inhale, and jump your feet about 4–4½ feet (1.3–1.5 meters) apart (depending on your stride) stretching your arms out at shoulder level. Adjust your feet until they are parallel, and stretch up.

2 Keeping your trunk facing forward, move your left foot slightly inward and rotate your right foot to the right, aligning the heel with your left instep.

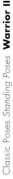

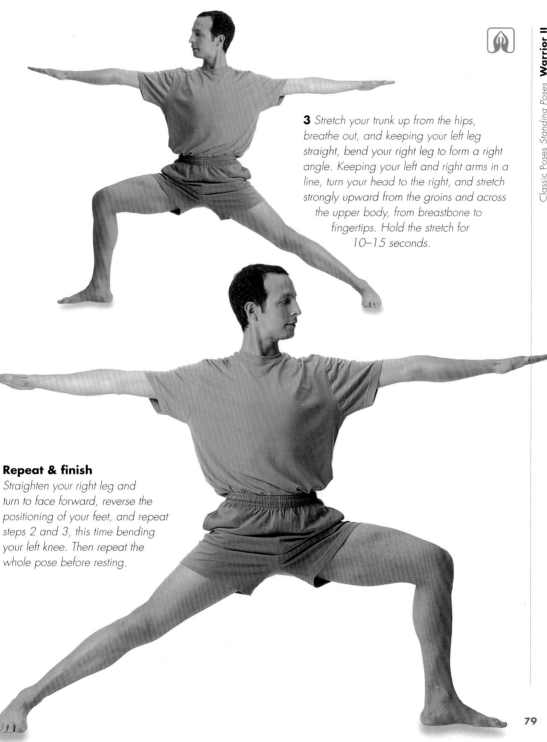

3 *Stretch your trunk up from the hips, breathe out, and keeping your left leg straight, bend your right leg to form a right angle. Keeping your left and right arms in a line, turn your head to the right, and stretch strongly upward from the groins and across the upper body, from breastbone to fingertips. Hold the stretch for 10–15 seconds.*

Repeat & finish

Straighten your right leg and turn to face forward, reverse the positioning of your feet, and repeat steps 2 and 3, this time bending your left knee. Then repeat the whole pose before resting.

79

Lifting & Stretching

I f you have worked through the ten poses in Chapter 3 once or twice, your legs should be stronger and your stance will be firmer. The two warrior poses—virabhadrasana II on pages 78–79, and the slightly more advanced virabhadrasana I on pages 82–85—work on strengthening the lower body. Focus your attention on maintaining an upward stretch and on the changing alignments of the different parts of your body. After jumping your legs apart in step 1, your feet must be parallel and the toes aligned so that your leg and foot face the same way.

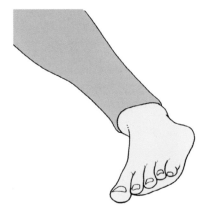

Working on the pose

Your stance needs to be firmly based, so when you turn your feet in step 2 the outer edge of the back foot must not lift, as shown above. If your weight is distributed evenly on both feet, the outer edge of the sole and heel rest firmly on the floor.

Your stance

At all stages of this pose keep your whole body lifted. Stand erect before you jump your legs apart, and pause before you rotate your feet to stretch your legs up from the arch of each foot to the hips. Turn each leg out at the hip joint, and lift your trunk from your groins. Keep your trunk erect as you bend your knee, and your head up.

If possible, check your stance at this stage in front of a mirror. The thigh of your bent leg should be parallel to the floor, and the shin needs to be at a 90° angle to the floor. Feel the stretch across your groins. While holding the pose, lift your breastbone and stretch out from the center of your chest. Extend your left arm to the left and your right arm to the right, keeping your shoulders down, then level your arms until they form a horizontal line across your body.

Points to Watch

- When your right knee is bent do not allow your left hip, the left side of your trunk, or your left shoulder to roll forward and down—and vice versa. Revolve them back as if pressing them against a wall.

- Keep your shoulders and your raised arm pressing back, so your arms and shoulders form a ruler-straight line.

- Keep your tailbone tucked in and your sitting bones stretching down.

Warrior II analyzed

To perfect your stance in step 3 of warrior II on page 79, check the details pinpointed on this image.

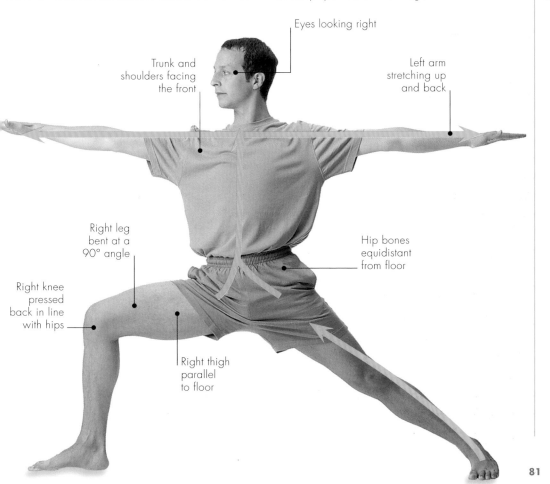

Eyes looking right

Trunk and shoulders facing the front

Left arm stretching up and back

Right leg bent at a 90° angle

Hip bones equidistant from floor

Right knee pressed back in line with hips

Right thigh parallel to floor

WARRIOR I

Virabhadrasana I is a strengthening pose, a dynamic posture in which you turn the trunk to the side. It stretches the joints between the vertebrae, working at restoring the spine's natural flexibility. It is recommended for its efficacy in relieving stiffness in the back, shoulders, and neck.

1 *Stand in tadasana, then inhale and jump your feet about 4–4½ feet (1.3–1.5 meters) apart depending on your stride, while stretching your arms out to shoulder level. Stretch upward and from fingertips to fingertips.*

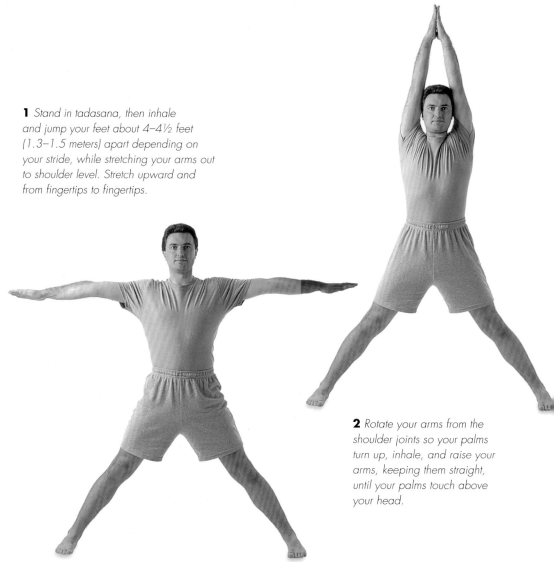

2 *Rotate your arms from the shoulder joints so your palms turn up, inhale, and raise your arms, keeping them straight, until your palms touch above your head.*

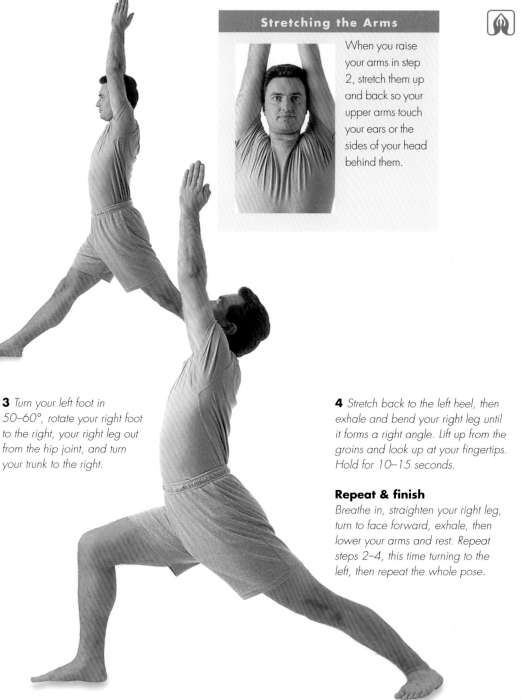

Stretching the Arms

When you raise your arms in step 2, stretch them up and back so your upper arms touch your ears or the sides of your head behind them.

3 Turn your left foot in 50–60°, rotate your right foot to the right, your right leg out from the hip joint, and turn your trunk to the right.

4 Stretch back to the left heel, then exhale and bend your right leg until it forms a right angle. Lift up from the groins and look up at your fingertips. Hold for 10–15 seconds.

Repeat & finish

Breathe in, straighten your right leg, turn to face forward, exhale, then lower your arms and rest. Repeat steps 2–4, this time turning to the left, then repeat the whole pose.

Arm Lifts

Warrior I is one of many poses that encourage you to flex, extend, and rotate your arms further than you thought they could go. You start the pose by extending your arms out at shoulder level, and stretching them. This stretch should be a powerful one, starting at the breastbone and flowing outward via the shoulder and the armpit, along each arm to the fingertips. In this pose you go further, however, rotating your outstretched arms backward through 180° from the shoulder joint until the palms face the ceiling, before raising your arms above your head.

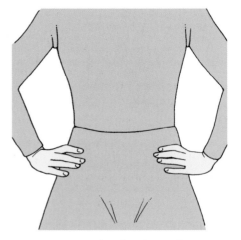

Preventing back strain
If you have a slipped disk or other more serious problem you should practice the pose without raising your arms above your head. If you keep your hands on your hips, you can work on your spine's flexibility without straining your back.

A powerful lift

The arm lift is a powerful movement that involves stretching more than just the arms. The stretch begins at the sides of the ribs, an action that lifts the rib cage, and stretches the armpits, the upper arms, the elbow joints, the forearms, and the hands. Work at stretching your upper arms all the way back to your ears—or even behind your ears—and bring your hands as close together as you can above your head, with your palms touching. This arm lift should be the culmination of a lifting movement that begins at the arch of the back foot, stretches up the inner back leg to the groins, rising to the hip bones and up the trunk to the neck and crown of the head. Finally, raise your head to look up at your outstretched hands with your fingertips touching.

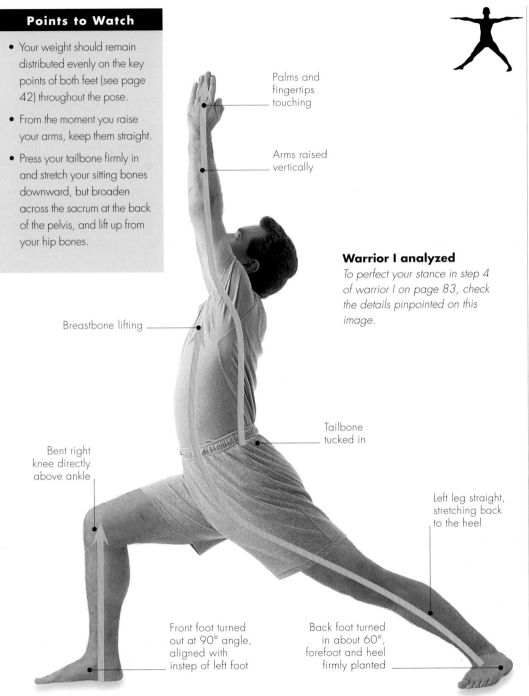

Points to Watch

- Your weight should remain distributed evenly on the key points of both feet (see page 42) throughout the pose.

- From the moment you raise your arms, keep them straight.

- Press your tailbone firmly in and stretch your sitting bones downward, but broaden across the sacrum at the back of the pelvis, and lift up from your hip bones.

Palms and fingertips touching

Arms raised vertically

Warrior I analyzed
To perfect your stance in step 4 of warrior I on page 83, check the details pinpointed on this image.

Breastbone lifting

Tailbone tucked in

Bent right knee directly above ankle

Left leg straight, stretching back to the heel

Front foot turned out at 90° angle, aligned with instep of left foot

Back foot turned in about 60°, forefoot and heel firmly planted

HALF MOON

The graceful **ardha chandrasana** pose is thought to resemble the half moon, hence its name. It radiates harmony, and it develops balance and coordination. All the standing poses strengthen the legs, but practiced regularly over time, this pose is especially beneficial for anyone with weak knees or ankles.

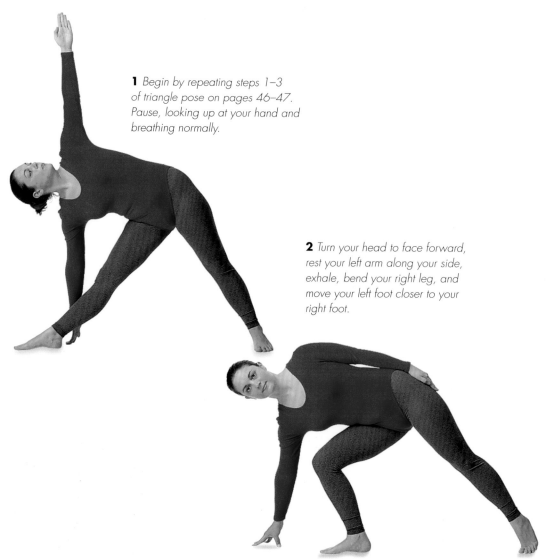

1 *Begin by repeating steps 1–3 of triangle pose on pages 46–47. Pause, looking up at your hand and breathing normally.*

2 *Turn your head to face forward, rest your left arm along your side, exhale, bend your right leg, and move your left foot closer to your right foot.*

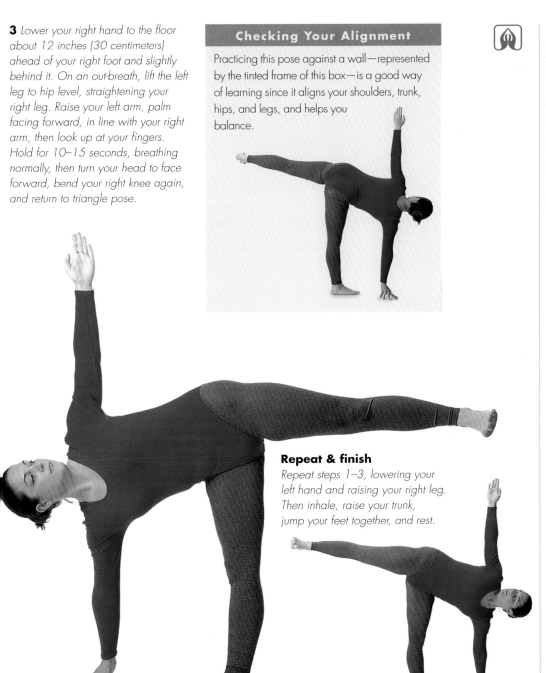

3 *Lower your right hand to the floor about 12 inches (30 centimeters) ahead of your right foot and slightly behind it. On an out-breath, lift the left leg to hip level, straightening your right leg. Raise your left arm, palm facing forward, in line with your right arm, then look up at your fingers. Hold for 10–15 seconds, breathing normally, then turn your head to face forward, bend your right knee again, and return to triangle pose.*

Checking Your Alignment

Practicing this pose against a wall—represented by the tinted frame of this box—is a good way of learning since it aligns your shoulders, trunk, hips, and legs, and helps you balance.

Repeat & finish
Repeat steps 1–3, lowering your left hand and raising your right leg. Then inhale, raise your trunk, jump your feet together, and rest.

Balance & Poise

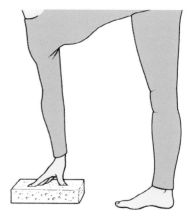

Half moon is a second-level asana which you begin in triangle pose (see pages 46–47), then balance on one hand and leg. Pause in triangle pose and concentrate on stretching and alignment. Breathe normally throughout, keeping both legs and both sides of your trunk stretching up.

Transferring your weight

Shifting your weight from two legs to one marks the transition from triangle to half moon in step 2. Make this transition smoothly, distributing your weight evenly onto the four key points on the sole of the foot (see page 42). As your left leg rises, you make another weight transfer onto your right leg. Turn your leg out from the hip as you raise it to hip level, so the knee faces forward.

Focus on balance

At this point, pause to balance yourself by stretching your standing leg strongly upward and your raised leg leftward, toward the outstretched foot. Fixing your gaze on your raised hand also helps you maintain your balance. The angle that is formed by your lower body is mirrored by

Working on the pose
If you cannot lower one hand right down to the floor, rest it on a pile of foam yoga blocks.

the upper body as you stretch your upper arm vertically in line with the downstretched arm. Here, pause to turn the entire upper side of your trunk up and back, and to press your tailbone in, then stretch your trunk from the groins to the crown of your head. Follow this movement by turning your head to look up, aligning it with your trunk.

Half moon analyzed

Step 3 of half moon pose on page 87 is detailed below. If you can, perform the pose in front of a mirror, checking each point shown.

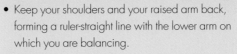

Points to Watch

- Keep your shoulders and your raised arm back, forming a ruler-straight line with the lower arm on which you are balancing.

- Do not allow the side of the trunk that is uppermost to roll forward. Revolve it back as if pressing it against a wall.

- Keep your tailbone tucked well in throughout the pose—do not allow your buttocks to protrude.

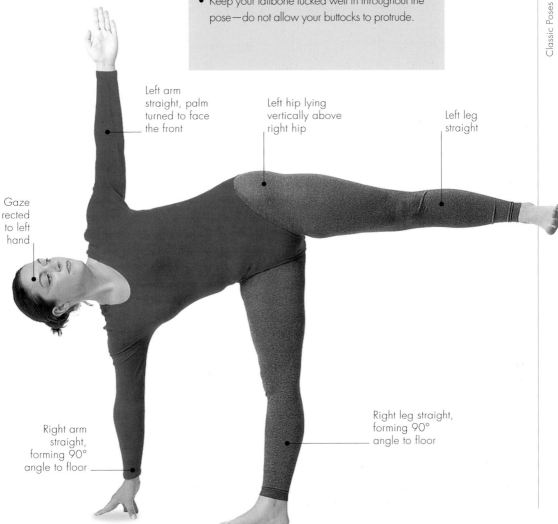

Left arm straight, palm turned to face the front

Left hip lying vertically above right hip

Left leg straight

Gaze rected to left hand

Right arm straight, forming 90° angle to floor

Right leg straight, forming 90° angle to floor

CHAIR

CHAIR **Utkatasana** is an antidote to the effects
of poor posture, because you sit in the air, balanced on
your two feet and using your own muscles for support.
Literally translated, the Sanskrit word "utkatasana" means
"powerful pose" and this is an apt description because it
gives power to the calves, the ankles, and the large
muscles of the buttocks and thighs.

Head & Arms

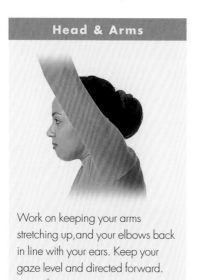

Work on keeping your arms
stretching up, and your elbows back
in line with your ears. Keep your
gaze level and directed forward.

1 *Stand in tadasana
(see page 43) with your
feet together, inhale,
raise your arms above
your head, and stretch up.*

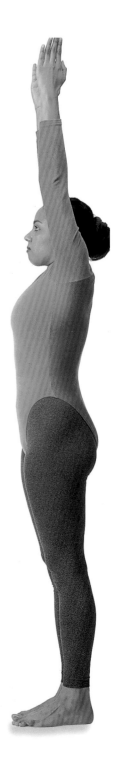

2 *On an out-breath, bend your ankles, your knees, and your hips, and lower your seat as if you were sitting on a chair, while keeping your heels on the floor. Hold for 10–15 seconds, stretching up from your hips.*

Hands & Arms

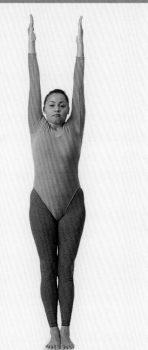

At first it is enough to raise your hands straight above your head as shown here, but as you progress, move your palms as close together as you can, until eventually your fingers and palms touch above your head.

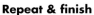

Repeat & finish
Straighten your legs and lower your arms to your sides. Stand briefly in tadasana, then repeat the pose.

Strengthening the Legs

The unusual positioning of the spine and pelvis in the chair pose on page 91 makes the muscles of the thighs, calves, and feet bear the weight of the upper body. It exercises the powerful, four-headed quadriceps muscle of the thigh, and exercises the calf muscles. Although we use these muscles when we sit, stand, run, and climb stairs, many of us neglect to stretch and exercise them, and our legs are often weaker than we think—as people often discover, painfully, after skiing practice. Chair pose is a great exercise for skiers and also for horse riders. It builds on the toning and strengthening you have already achieved by practicing standing poses.

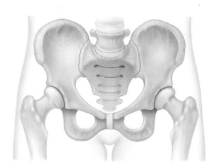

Aligning the pelvis

Do not tuck your tailbone under but imagine you are stretching the sacrum and sitting bones at the base of the pelvis down to the floor Simultaneously lift the hip bones at the front.

Forming diagonals

In this pose, the arms, trunk, thighs, and calves form a succession of diagonals. Because the body is bent into a sitting position, the trunk inclines along a diagonal, but in fact the spine is straight. The chair depends on the correct alignment of the pelvic girdle, which must not be tucked right in and under, nor pushed out behind. If you find your lower body is stiff when you try the pose, move your feet about 12 inches (30 centimeters) apart at the beginning of step 1. The stretching action of the raised arms is an excellent exercise for the shoulders, an area of the body that is often found to be stiff.

Points to Watch

- Keep your shoulders and hips in horizontal alignment.

- Let the trunk incline forward from the hips, but keep your back straight and stretching up.

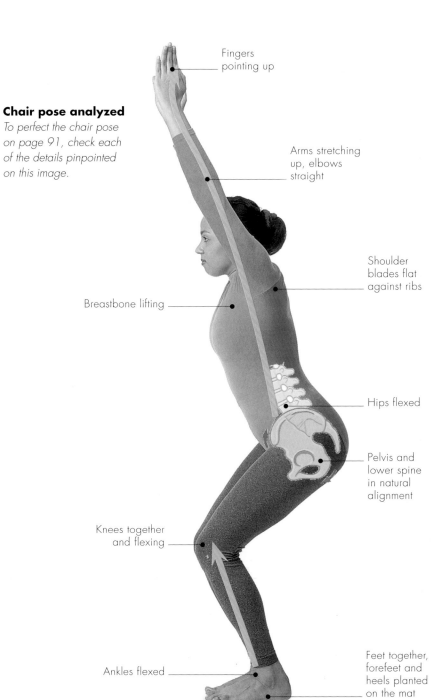

Fingers
pointing up

Arms stretching
up, elbows
straight

Chair pose analyzed
*To perfect the chair pose
on page 91, check each
of the details pinpointed
on this image.*

Shoulder
blades flat
against ribs

Breastbone lifting

Hips flexed

Pelvis and
lower spine
in natural
alignment

Knees together
and flexing

Feet together,
forefeet and
heels planted
on the mat

Ankles flexed

SIDE-STRETCH

A forward bend that extends the legs is a good pose to follow the bent-legged chair pose on the preceding pages. In **parsvottanasana** the body extends over one forward-striding leg. This pose is really two exercises in one, since the arms join behind the back in **namaste**, the prayer pose.

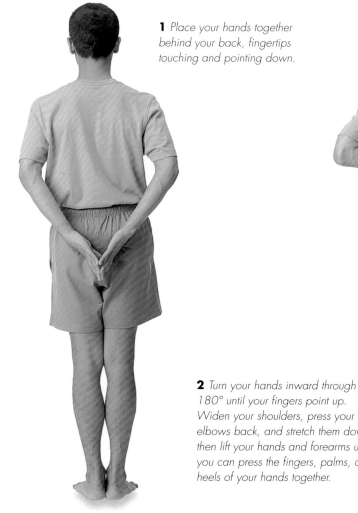

1 *Place your hands together behind your back, fingertips touching and pointing down.*

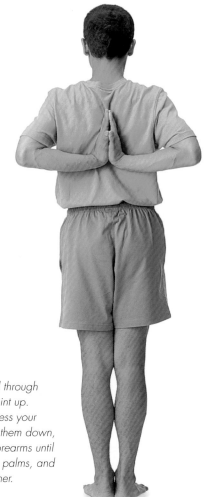

2 *Turn your hands inward through 180° until your fingers point up. Widen your shoulders, press your elbows back, and stretch them down, then lift your hands and forearms until you can press the fingers, palms, and heels of your hands together.*

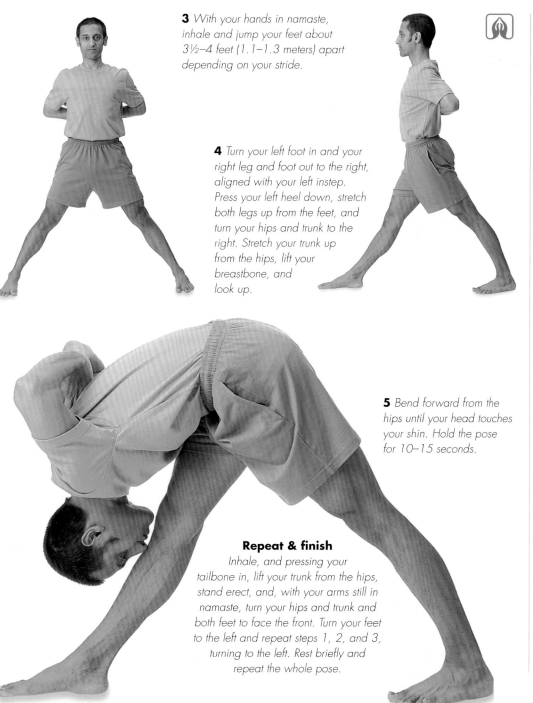

3 With your hands in namaste, inhale and jump your feet about 3½–4 feet (1.1–1.3 meters) apart depending on your stride.

4 Turn your left foot in and your right leg and foot out to the right, aligned with your left instep. Press your left heel down, stretch both legs up from the feet, and turn your hips and trunk to the right. Stretch your trunk up from the hips, lift your breastbone, and look up.

5 Bend forward from the hips until your head touches your shin. Hold the pose for 10–15 seconds.

Repeat & finish
Inhale, and pressing your tailbone in, lift your trunk from the hips, stand erect, and, with your arms still in namaste, turn your hips and trunk and both feet to face the front. Turn your feet to the left and repeat steps 1, 2, and 3, turning to the left. Rest briefly and repeat the whole pose.

Intensive Stretching

This standing pose gives the body a strong stretch—its Sanskrit name, parsvottanasana, means "intensive stretching." As you bend to the right, you stretch the muscles and joints of the legs, the knee and hip joints, and sides of the abdomen and chest. At the same time the prayer position of the hands activates the pectoral muscles of the upper chest and arms and the muscles that move both the shoulders and the collar bone.

Hand position

This pose incorporates a special hand position—namaste, the prayer pose, which is more familiar when performed at the front rather than the back of the body. You may need to first practice rotating the wrist to turn the downward-pointing hands, fingertips touching behind your back, inward and up. With your fingers pointing towards the ceiling, widen your shoulders and press your forearms back, stretching the elbows down. This will help you raise your forearms and joined hands behind your back—and you will find that the higher you raise them, stretching up as you do so, the more your chest opens. With practice you will be able to press not only your fingers together but also the palms, the thumbs, and the heels of your hands.

Upward stretch

Strong legs are the foundation of forward bends, so before bending forward, take a moment to stretch from feet to head. Lift the arches of your feet and feel an upward stretch in both legs—but more of a stretch in the back leg because you press the outer edge of the heel firmly down. Check that one hip is not positioned higher or further forward than the other, and keep the wings of your arms stretching firmly back. Lift your trunk up from your hip bones, raising your breastbone as you look up.

As you bend forward from the hips, extend your trunk away from your legs. Feel the intense stretch from your legs along your sides. This mobilizes the hip joints, and, incidentally, has the effect of flattening the lower abdomen, in addition to giving the lungs more breathing space.

Side-stretches analyzed

When you have mastered the hand position, work on the points shown here to perfect the side-stretch on page 95.

Upper arms stretching back toward hips

Hands pressed together, fingertips pointing to head

Hips bending, hip bones level

Legs turned out at hip joints

Head touching shin, neck relaxed

WIDE LEG-STRETCH
Stretching the legs very wide apart exercises the abductor muscles of the hips. These rotate the legs outward from the center of the body and are often underused. **Prasarita padottanasana** increases blood circulation through the trunk and to the head, and it is said to help if you are trying to slim your hips.

1 *Stand in tadasana (see page 43), stretch your arms out to shoulder level, inhale, and jump the feet about 4½–5 feet (1.5–1.7 meters) apart, or as wide as your stride allows. Align your toes and turn both feet in slightly.*

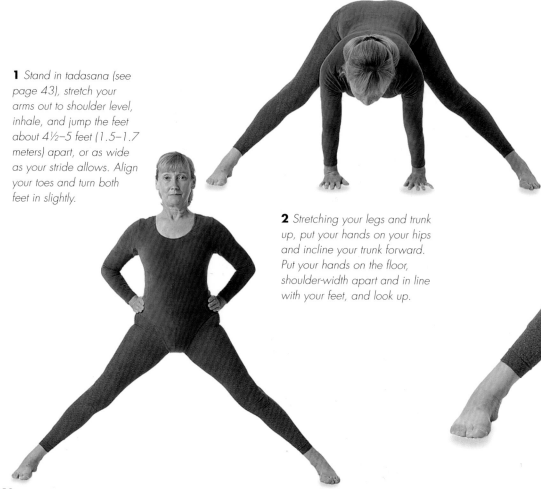

2 *Stretching your legs and trunk up, put your hands on your hips and incline your trunk forward. Put your hands on the floor, shoulder-width apart and in line with your feet, and look up.*

3 *Stretch your spine forward, breathe out, bend your elbows, and keeping them parallel, lower the crown of your head to the mat between your hands. Hold the pose for 10–15 seconds, keeping your elbows in.*

Repeat & finish

Raise your head, straighten your arms, breathe in, straighten your back, and stand up. Breathe out, jump your feet together, rest, and repeat the pose.

Downward Stretch

Lift your trunk from the hips before bending forward in step 2, and bend from the hips. Straighten your spine and lift your breast-bone before stretching down in step 3.

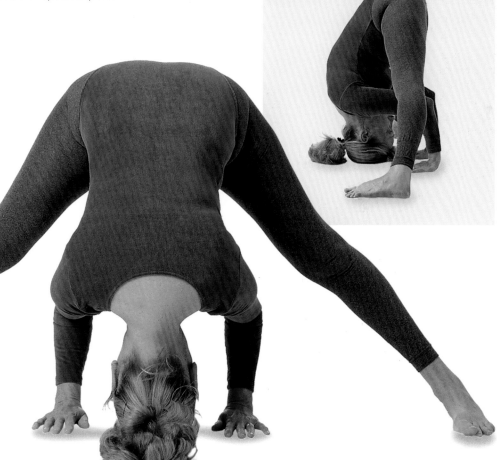

Loosening the Hamstrings

Like many people, you may find your hips bend easily when you try the wide leg-stretch on pages 98–99, but that you need to work on your legs. Most dancers will find this pose easy because the hips incline forward readily if the hamstrings are flexible. Try the pose and if you cannot reach the floor, rest your hands on a pile of foam yoga blocks, or on the seat of a chair with its back against a wall.

Preparation

As you jump your feet apart at the start, distribute your body weight evenly on the four key points of both feet, then lift your arches and your ankles so they do not sag outward, and stretch your legs up. Keep your legs stretching up, your arms and your spine straight, and your breastbone lifting as you lift your head and look up in step 2.

Semimembrinosus   Semitendinosus

Biceps femoris

The hamstrings
Three muscles with long names stretch down the back of the thigh. They straighten it and bend and rotate the knee. Two have long sheaths and tendons (the "hamstrings"), which attach them to the bones of the pelvis.

Working on the hamstrings

Your legs need to be pressing back as well as lifting throughout this pose, and you should feel a strong stretch from feet to hips. If your hamstrings are tight they will quickly loosen with practice and you can gradually reduce the number of foam yoga blocks you are using for support. Eventually, your legs will be flexible enough to allow you to lower your hands, and eventually your head, to the mat.

Points to Watch

- Do not curve your back into a hump when you bend from the hips in step 2. Your spine should be slightly concave (inward-curving).

- In step 3 keep your elbows parallel and drawn in toward your chest. Do not let them stick out from your body like wings.

- When you lower your head to the floor, keep your weight on your feet by stretching your legs up and keeping your hips and heels in line.

Wide leg-stretch analyzed

Achieving the full wide leg-stretch in step 3 on page 99 takes regular practice and careful attention to the details shown here.

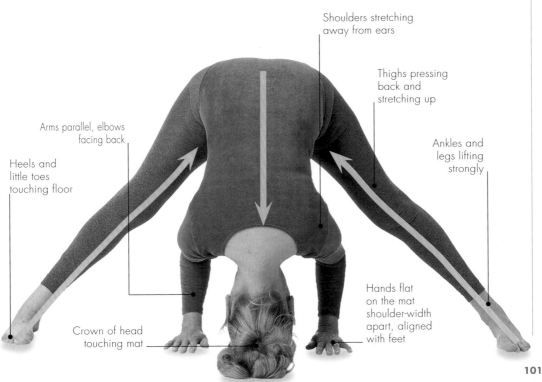

Shoulders stretching away from ears

Thighs pressing back and stretching up

Arms parallel, elbows facing back

Heels and little toes touching floor

Ankles and legs lifting strongly

Crown of head touching mat

Hands flat on the mat shoulder-width apart, aligned with feet

REVOLVED TRIANGLE Parivrtta trikonasana is a standing twist

in which you begin with your trunk facing forward and you end up with it facing the opposite direction—so it is often called "reverse triangle." It is the last of the sequence of standing poses which begin this chapter.

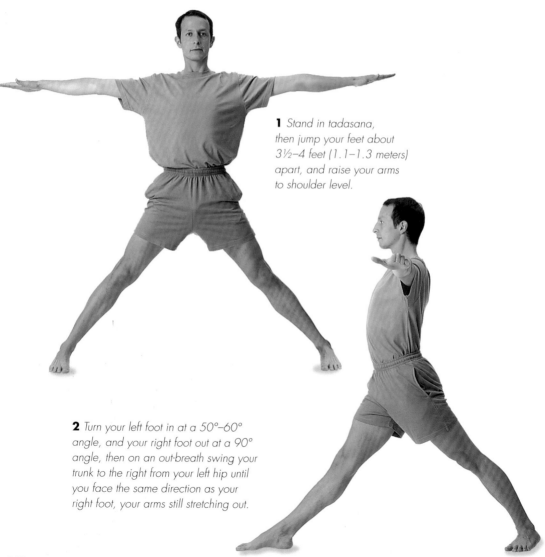

1 *Stand in tadasana, then jump your feet about 3½–4 feet (1.1–1.3 meters) apart, and raise your arms to shoulder level.*

2 *Turn your left foot in at a 50°–60° angle, and your right foot out at a 90° angle, then on an out-breath swing your trunk to the right from your left hip until you face the same direction as your right foot, your arms still stretching out.*

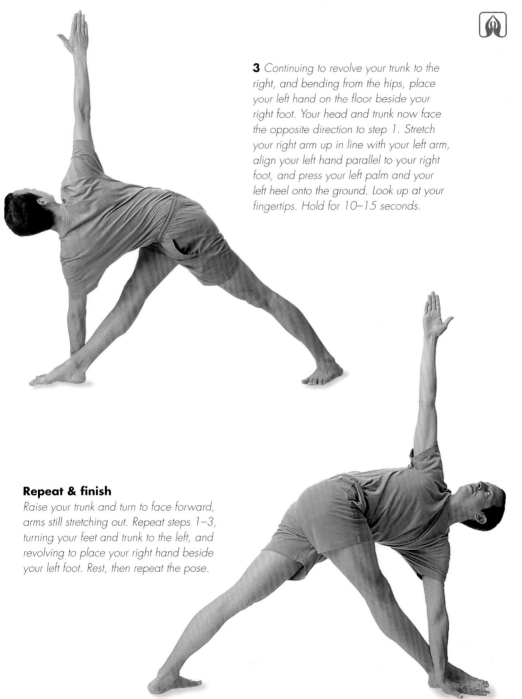

3 *Continuing to revolve your trunk to the right, and bending from the hips, place your left hand on the floor beside your right foot. Your head and trunk now face the opposite direction to step 1. Stretch your right arm up in line with your left arm, align your left hand parallel to your right foot, and press your left palm and your left heel onto the ground. Look up at your fingertips. Hold for 10–15 seconds.*

Repeat & finish

Raise your trunk and turn to face forward, arms still stretching out. Repeat steps 1–3, turning your feet and trunk to the left, and revolving to place your right hand beside your left foot. Rest, then repeat the pose.

Turning the Trunk

For the triangle pose on pages 46–49 your trunk remains facing forward while you bend to left or right, placing one hand on the floor beside the front foot. In the revolved triangle on pages 102–103 you turn the trunk through a half circle before you bend it and rest your hand on the mat. The pose gives the spine a satisfying twist.

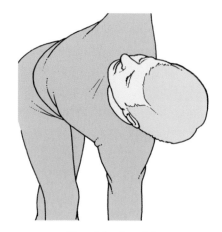

Head & shoulders
Keep your shoulders back and your shoulder blades flat against your ribs. Straighten your spine and align your head with it so that neck and head lie at right angles to your shoulders.

Which way to turn?

You began facing forward, but as you revolve your trunk, your head turns with it, so you look backward. Practicing close to a wall makes it easier to work out which way to turn. Begin facing the wall, and turn your trunk until you face into the room. Stretch your legs up and your arms out before twisting your trunk, and breathe in. Turn on the out-breath, rotating the hips, the abdomen, the waist, and the chest.

Stretching your spine away from your legs helps you turn and bend further. If your spine needs more flexibility, lower your hand onto a chair seat, then progress down to a pile of telephone books placed beside your little toe. Pause to equalize your weight on the four key points on each foot. Stretch both legs up from the arches of your feet, and press the palm and heel of your downward-stretching hand flat on the floor beside what is now your front foot. As you turn your face up, check that your upward-stretching arm rises vertically from your shoulders, so your outstretched arms form a straight line. Breathe normally as you hold the pose.

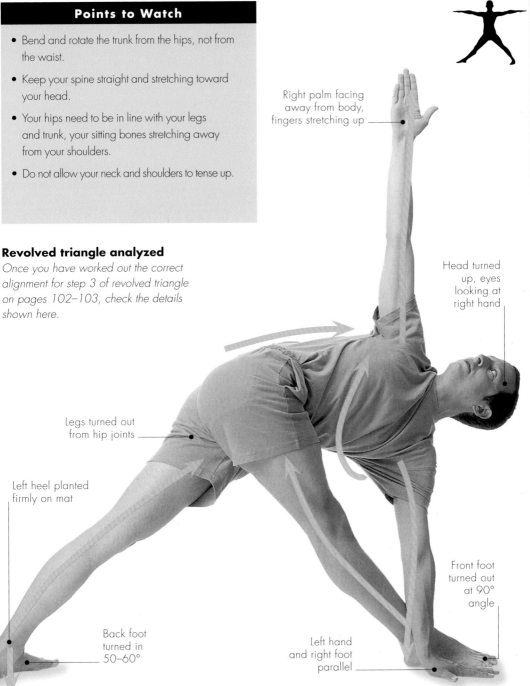

Points to Watch

- Bend and rotate the trunk from the hips, not from the waist.

- Keep your spine straight and stretching toward your head.

- Your hips need to be in line with your legs and trunk, your sitting bones stretching away from your shoulders.

- Do not allow your neck and shoulders to tense up.

Revolved triangle analyzed

Once you have worked out the correct alignment for step 3 of revolved triangle on pages 102–103, check the details shown here.

Right palm facing away from body, fingers stretching up

Head turned up, eyes looking at right hand

Legs turned out from hip joints

Left heel planted firmly on mat

Back foot turned in 50–60°

Left hand and right foot parallel

Front foot turned out at 90° angle

SITTING & KNEELING

This page begins a sequence of sitting poses, starting with rod pose or **dandasana**, which is the foundation of most sitting asanas, and hero pose, **virasana**, which underlies all kneeling postures. These asanas rest the heart, quiet the mind, and calm the nerves. They are an antidote to stress and encourage a good night's sleep.

Rod pose

Sit on a mat, stretch your legs out, and place your hands on the floor either side of your hips. Press your hands and legs down and stretch up from your hips. Hold the stretch for 15–20 seconds, then rest.

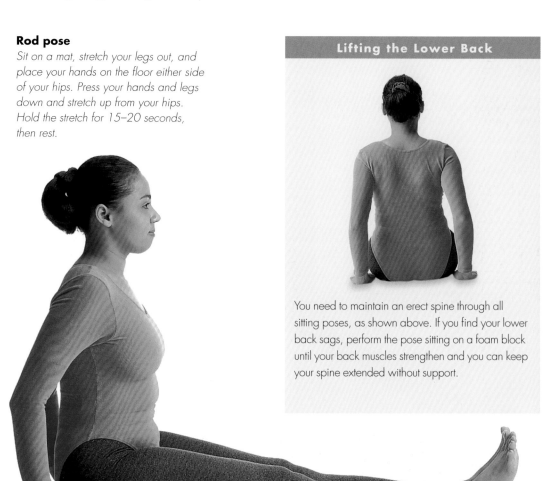

Lifting the Lower Back

You need to maintain an erect spine through all sitting poses, as shown above. If you find your lower back sags, perform the pose sitting on a foam block until your back muscles strengthen and you can keep your spine extended without support.

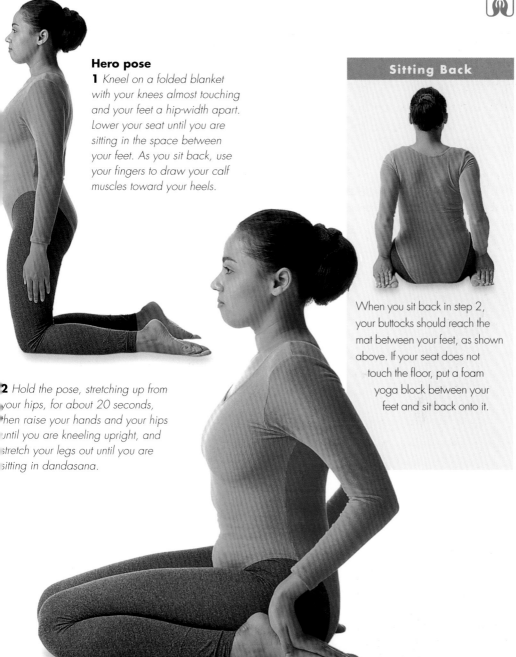

Hero pose

1 *Kneel on a folded blanket with your knees almost touching and your feet a hip-width apart. Lower your seat until you are sitting in the space between your feet. As you sit back, use your fingers to draw your calf muscles toward your heels.*

2 *Hold the pose, stretching up from your hips, for about 20 seconds, then raise your hands and your hips until you are kneeling upright, and stretch your legs out until you are sitting in dandasana.*

Sitting Back

When you sit back in step 2, your buttocks should reach the mat between your feet, as shown above. If your seat does not touch the floor, put a foam yoga block between your feet and sit back onto it.

Basic Floor Work

Dandasana is called rod pose because the back must be rod-straight and stretching up. Sitting on a foam block or a blanket folded two or three times will help, and as you lower your buttocks to the floor pull the large gluteal muscles that form the fleshy buttocks out to the sides. Then, to help yourself lift your trunk you need to press your legs into the floor and use the rebound to stretch up from the hips.

Kneeling

In virasana, the hero pose, you kneel, but sit between widely parted feet. It is good for stiff knees, but if when you sit back your buttocks do not reach the floor your legs tend to roll inward. This stretches the knees unevenly, causing discomfort.

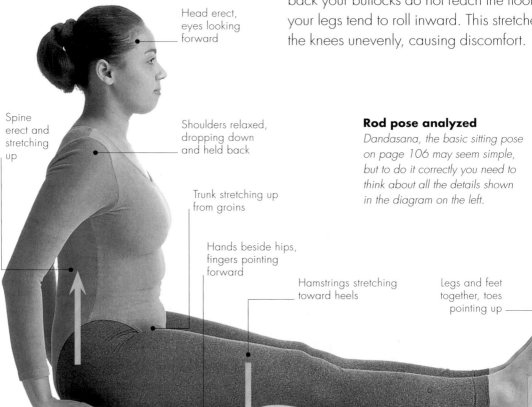

Head erect, eyes looking forward

Spine erect and stretching up

Shoulders relaxed, dropping down and held back

Trunk stretching up from groins

Hands beside hips, fingers pointing forward

Hamstrings stretching toward heels

Legs and feet together, toes pointing up

Rod pose analyzed
Dandasana, the basic sitting pose on page 106 may seem simple, but to do it correctly you need to think about all the details shown in the diagram on the left.

Placing a foam block between your feet will help you to keep your thighs aligned and to maintain an erect back while stretching up from the hips. If your knees or your feet are painful at first, place a small folded towel or blanket at the back of each knee, or beneath your ankles and feet.

Hero pose analyzed

Checking the details shown in the illustration on the right will help you perfect the hero pose or virasana on page 107.

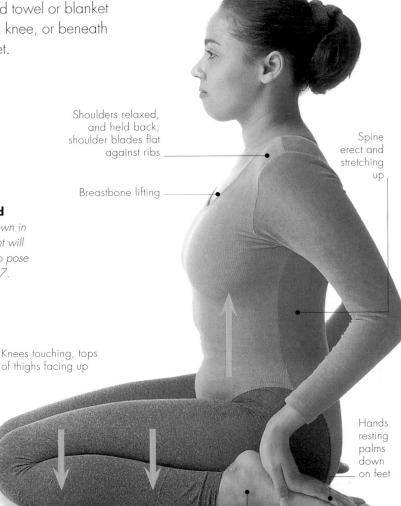

Shoulders relaxed, and held back, shoulder blades flat against ribs

Breastbone lifting

Spine erect and stretching up

Knees touching, tops of thighs facing up

Hands resting palms down on feet

Insteps touching hips, toes pointing back

ANGLED LEG POSES

Baddha konasana is often called cobbler pose because in India cobblers traditionally work sitting with their knees wide apart and their feet together. Sitting with the legs widely angled, as in cobbler pose and the angled leg-stretch, **upavistha konasana**, gives a good stretch across the groins. They are believed to be effective in preventing urinary disorders and relieving menstrual pains.

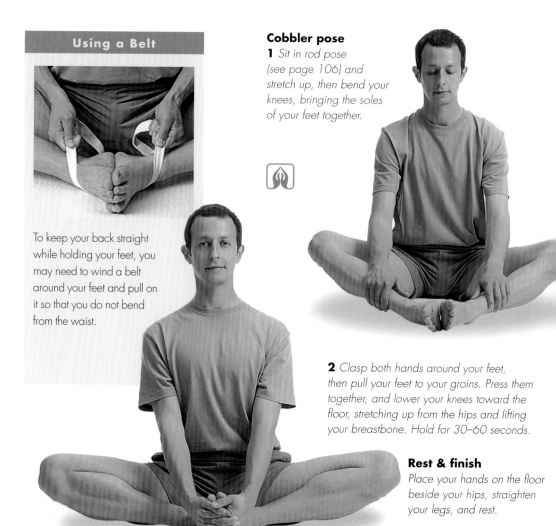

Using a Belt

To keep your back straight while holding your feet, you may need to wind a belt around your feet and pull on it so that you do not bend from the waist.

Cobbler pose

1 *Sit in rod pose (see page 106) and stretch up, then bend your knees, bringing the soles of your feet together.*

2 *Clasp both hands around your feet, then pull your feet to your groins. Press them together, and lower your knees toward the floor, stretching up from the hips and lifting your breastbone. Hold for 30–60 seconds.*

Rest & finish

Place your hands on the floor beside your hips, straighten your legs, and rest.

Angled leg-stretch

1 *Sit in rod pose and stretch up, then keeping your back straight and your toes pointing up, move your legs out as far as you comfortably can so they form a wide angle. Press your hands and legs into the floor and stretch up, then, on an out-breath, bend your trunk forward from the hips, stretching your arms out, and catch hold of your big toes. Hold for 5–10 seconds.*

2 *On an out-breath, pull on your toes, and stretch forward and as far down as you can—if possible, until your forehead touches the floor. Hold the stretch for 5–10 seconds.*

Rest & finish
Breathe in, raise your head and your trunk, place your hands on the mat beside your hips, move your legs together, and rest.

Warning

If your legs feel strained when you catch hold of your toes in step 1, do not go on to step 2. Instead, breathe in, move your legs together, and rest. Return to this pose later, when your back and hips have become more flexible.

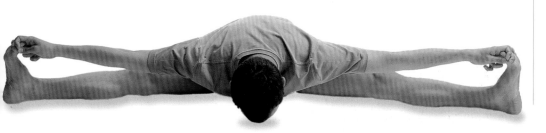

Stretching the Hip Joints

The two leg-stretches on pages 110–11 involve flexing the hips as well as stretching across the groins. In the angled leg-stretch you incline the spine forward as far as you can without bending from the waist. This movement exercises the lumbar spine, the hip joints, and the muscles and tendons of the buttocks and thighs. And in the cobbler pose you lower your bent knees to the floor while keeping your back straight.

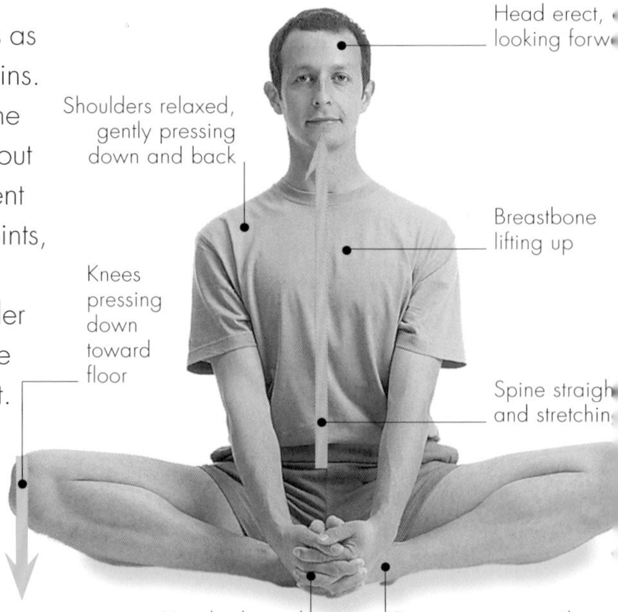
Head erect,
Shoulders relaxed, gently pressing down and back
Breastbone lifting up
Knees pressing down toward floor
Hands clasped around feet
Feet pressing together and in toward groins

Cobbler pose analyzed

The diagram on the right shows a number of important details to check in step 2 of the cobbler pose on page 110.

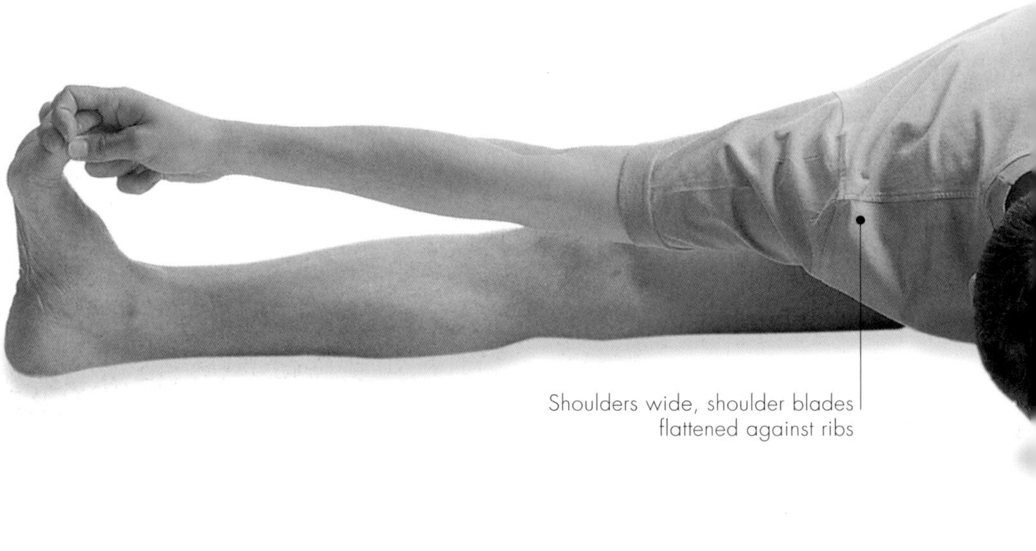
Shoulders wide, shoulder blades flattened against ribs

Aids to stretching

Begin both poses by sitting in the rod pose on a folded blanket or a foam yoga block. This makes it easier to lift the lower back, and in the cobbler pose helps you lower your knees to the floor. If your knees are high off the floor at first, sit on three folded blankets or two foam blocks.

If when you bend forward in the angled leg-stretch your hands do not reach your toes, do not allow yourself to bend from the waist, but instead work on your hip flexion by holding on to your calves. And if at first you cannot stretch down far enough to touch your forehead to the mat, rest it on a foam block, or on the seat of a chair positioned in front of you. Eventually, with practice, you will be able to extend your trunk further forward and rest your forehead on the mat in the full pose.

Angled leg-stretch analyzed
Check you have the details shown below correct when you practice the full angled leg-stretch on page 111.

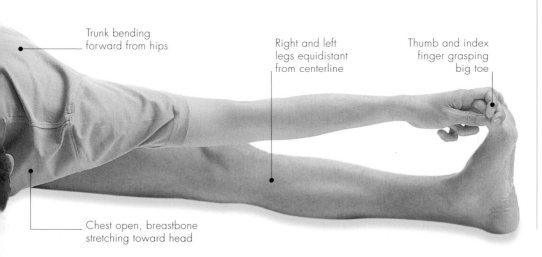

Trunk bending forward from hips

Right and left legs equidistant from centerline

Thumb and index finger grasping big toe

Chest open, breastbone stretching toward head

HEAD-TO-KNEE

The head-to-knee pose or **janu sirsasana** is a forward bend from a sitting position. It stimulates the organs of digestion, particularly the liver and kidneys, and is said to be particularly helpful to men with prostate disorders. Like all forward bends, it is a restful, calming posture.

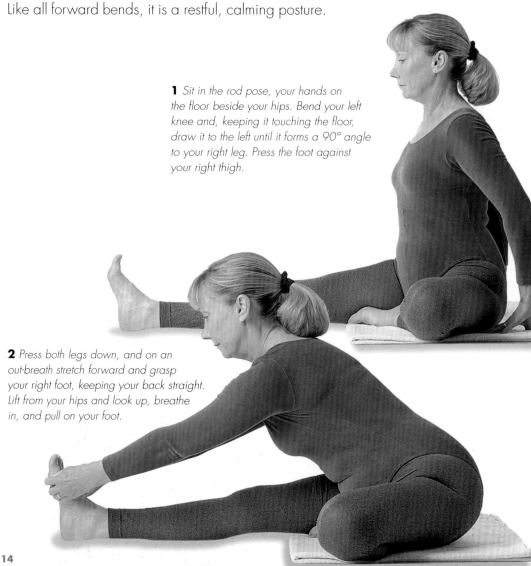

1 *Sit in the rod pose, your hands on the floor beside your hips. Bend your left knee and, keeping it touching the floor, draw it to the left until it forms a 90° angle to your right leg. Press the foot against your right thigh.*

2 *Press both legs down, and on an out-breath stretch forward and grasp your right foot, keeping your back straight. Lift from your hips and look up, breathe in, and pull on your foot.*

Relaxing into the Pose

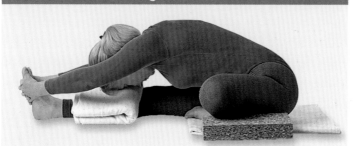

If your bent knee is uncomfortable, rest it on a foam block or a folded blanket. Your head and neck need to be relaxed, so if your forehead does not reach your shin, rest it on a blanket folded three or four times, or on a foam block.

Repeat & finish
Release your foot, stretch out your left leg, inhale, and raise your head and trunk until you are sitting in the rod pose. Then repeat steps 1–3, bending your right leg.

3 *On the out-breath, extend your trunk along your right leg, resting your forehead on the shin. Hold the extension for 10–15 seconds, breathing normally.*

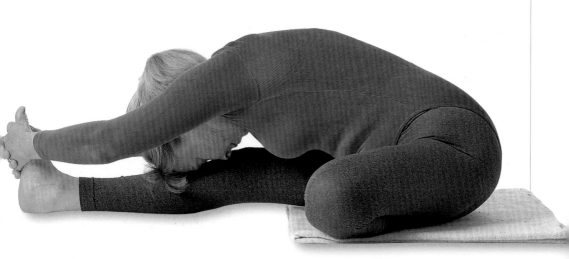

Straightening the Spine

All the sitting forward bends begin in the rod pose, and they depend on stretching the back until it is as straight as possible. Even when bending forward to touch your knee with your head in janu sirsasana on pages 114–15 you need to elongate your trunk, lifting from your hips, and extending forward from the groins. If you bend from your waist you will find it hard to straighten your trunk, so your hands may not reach your feet. Use each opportunity the pose provides to stretch your spine from your fifth lumbar vertebra to the atlas on which your skull rests, and your trunk from groins to breastbone.

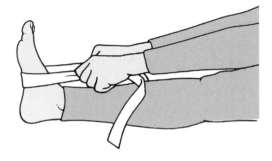

Working on the pose
Work on bending from the hips by winding a belt round your outstretched foot, holding one side of the belt in each hand, and pulling on it. Press your foot into the belt as you walk your hands down it, right, then left, then right.

Achieving the stretch

In step 2, press your legs down in order to stretch up further before lowering your head to your outstretched leg in step 3. If you can reach your foot, hold it in both hands, and pull on it to lever your trunk forward, but do not strain your body in trying to reach it. Instead, use a belt to pull your trunk forward as shown in the illustration above, while keeping your spine straight and stretching, and inclining your trunk a little further forward each time a hand moves forward. If at first your head does not reach your leg, place a folded blanket or a foam block on your shin and rest it on that—and put one under your bent knee if it feels uncomfortable. As you practice, your body becomes more flexible, until eventually you can clasp your hands around your foot and relax down into the full pose, resting your forehead on your leg.

Points to Watch

- When you bend your leg in step 1, draw the foot toward the opposite leg until it just rests against the groin and the top of the thigh. Be careful not to push it under the outstretched leg or beneath the thigh.

- Stretch your trunk toward your head, keeping your chest parallel with the floor and your breastbone in line with your straight leg.

Head-to-knee pose analyzed

Observing each of the details pinpointed on the image below will help you achieve the full head-to-knee pose on page 115.

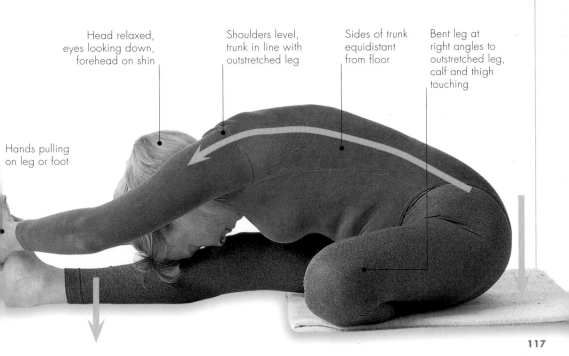

Head relaxed, eyes looking down, forehead on shin

Shoulders level, trunk in line with outstretched leg

Sides of trunk equidistant from floor

Bent leg at right angles to outstretched leg, calf and thigh touching

Hands pulling on leg or foot

THREE-LIMBED POSE

The body is said to have three limbs in this pose: the feet, the knees, and the buttocks. Its lengthy Sanskrit name—**triang mukhaikapada paschimottanasana**—indicates that in this forward bend the head touches one leg. This pose stimulates the digestive system and relaxes the heart and brain, and is said to relieve pain and swelling in the legs and feet.

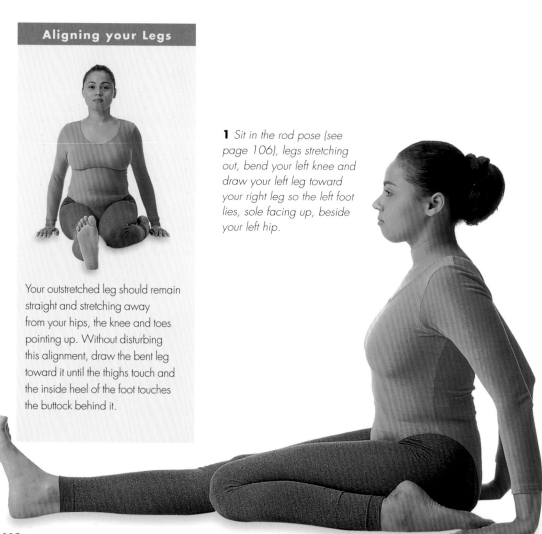

Aligning your Legs

Your outstretched leg should remain straight and stretching away from your hips, the knee and toes pointing up. Without disturbing this alignment, draw the bent leg toward it until the thighs touch and the inside heel of the foot touches the buttock behind it.

1 *Sit in the rod pose (see page 106), legs stretching out, bend your left knee and draw your left leg toward your right leg so the left foot lies, sole facing up, beside your left hip.*

2 *Press both legs down, lift your spine, and on an out-breath stretch forward and catch hold of your foot. Extend your trunk forward from the hips along the outstretched leg until your forehead touches the shin. Hold for about 20 seconds.*

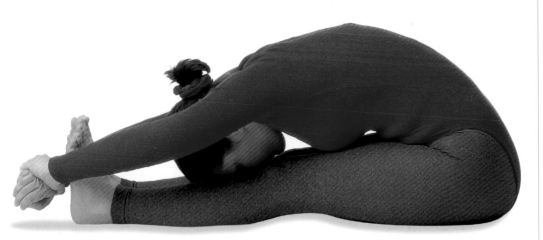

Leveling Your Pelvis

Keep your pelvis level. Your hip bones should remain aligned when you bend your leg in step 1, and both sitting bones should press down to the floor through the pose.

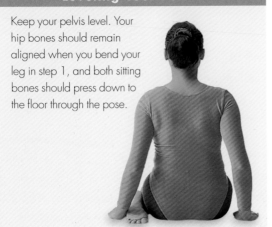

Repeat & finish

Lift your head, stretch and straighten your spine, release your hands, and raise your trunk until you sit in the rod pose. Then repeat steps 1 and 2, this time bending your right leg.

Working the Legs & Feet

The legs and feet are often over-used but underexercised, and the three-limbed pose on pages 118–19 helps to redress the balance. Each leg is bent and stretched in turn, exercising the knee joint, stretching and flexing the ankle joint, and strengthening the arches of the feet. Stretching each extended leg toward the foot while pressing it down exercises the hamstrings and the quadriceps muscles of the thighs, and the calf muscles.

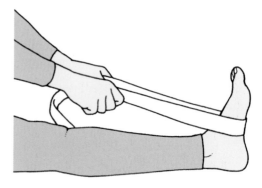

Using a belt

Wind a belt around the sole of your foot, hold one end in each hand, stretch your spine up, and pull on the belt with your hands while pressing into it with your foot to bend forward from the hips.

Three limbs

The third limb in this three-limbed pose is held to be the seat, and this stresses the active role of the hips in forward bends. Begin this posture sitting in the rod pose, with your hips level, and press equally down on both sitting bones as you bend your leg and incline your trunk forward. If you find that it is difficult to keep your hips level during this action, raise the level of your pelvis by sitting on a folded blanket or a foam block.

While the head-to-knee pose on pages 114–15 works the abductors—the muscles that turn the leg out at the hip— this pose exercises the adductors. These muscles turn the leg in toward the body's midline. Use them to keep your thighs parallel and pressing down, the centerline of both pointing up.

Press your hips and both legs down and lift your trunk before stretching forward. If your hands only reach your outstretched calf, use a belt as illustrated. And if your head does not reach your shin, rest it on a pillow or even on a chair seat.

Persevering with the three-limbed pose improves the mobility of your hip joints, and with practice you will soon be able to clasp your hands behind your foot without difficulty.

Points to Watch

- Keep your balance—the center of each thigh needs to face the ceiling throughout.

- Pull on your foot to lever your body forward, bending your elbows and keeping them the same distance from the floor.

- Stretch the front of your body, from pelvis to breastbone, as well as your back.

Three-limbed pose analyzed

It is essential to position the parts of the body accurately in yoga, so check the details pinpointed below for step 2 of the three-limbed pose on page 119.

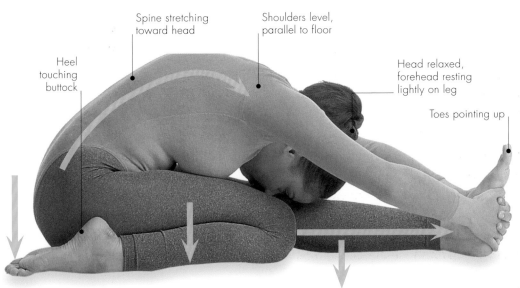

Spine stretching toward head

Shoulders level, parallel to floor

Heel touching buttock

Head relaxed, forehead resting lightly on leg

Toes pointing up

SITTING FORWARD BEND

In this forward bend, called **paschimottanasana**, you extend your whole body forward from the hips as if you were folding yourself in half. By positioning the heart below the spine, it reduces the heart's workload and stretches the spine, increasing the circulation to the lower body, so it calms, relaxes, refreshes, and revitalizes.

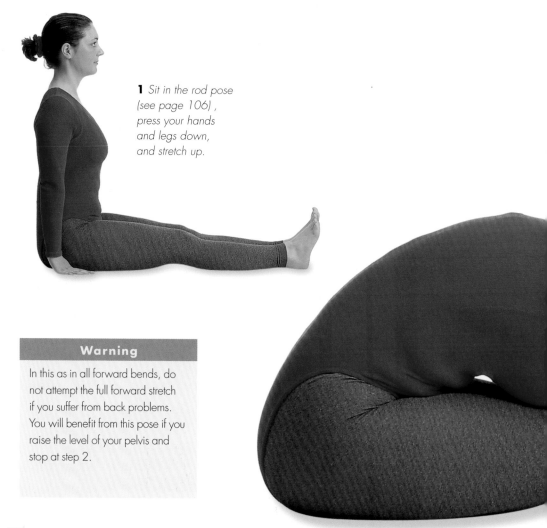

1 *Sit in the rod pose (see page 106), press your hands and legs down, and stretch up.*

Warning

In this as in all forward bends, do not attempt the full forward stretch if you suffer from back problems. You will benefit from this pose if you raise the level of your pelvis and stop at step 2.

2 *On an out-breath and bending from the hips, stretch your arms forward and catch hold of the sides of your feet, straightening your spine.*

Working on the Pose

Do not bend at the waist in the effort to reach your feet. Instead, wind a belt around the soles of your feet and walk your hands down it as far as you can, stretching a little further forward from the hips each time you move your hands along the belt.

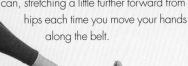

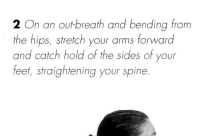

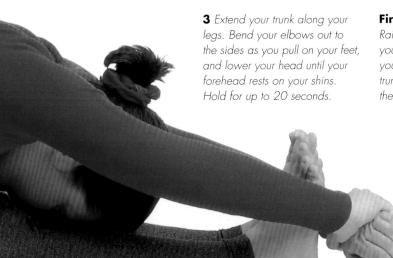

3 *Extend your trunk along your legs. Bend your elbows out to the sides as you pull on your feet, and lower your head until your forehead rests on your shins. Hold for up to 20 seconds.*

Finish & rest
Raise your head, release your hands, and keeping your back straight, raise your trunk until you are sitting in the rod pose, then rest.

An Extreme Stretch

The sitting forward bend on pages 122–23 ends a sequence of three forward bends, giving the body the most intense stretch of all. Unless your back is very supple and your hip joints flexible, you may need to work on the pose for some time before you can achieve it without using aids. If you can reach forward only as far as your knees or calves, begin by sitting on a foam block or folded blankets and use a belt to pull your trunk forward while keeping your back as straight as you can. You might begin practicing by placing a low chair over your outstretched legs and resting your forehead on the seat, or placing one or more foam blocks on your knees. As your body develops flexibility, the forward bend will become easier.

The impetus to stretch

Stretching up from the hips makes it easier to bend from the hips. It also elongates the spine, enabling you to reach further. It is easy in a demanding pose to let your trunk sag backward, so pause from time to time and press your sitting bones, your legs, and your feet down onto the floor firmly, to give yourself the impetus to stretch your spine and breastbone toward your head. Grasp your feet, stretching your elbows out to either side—or pull on the belt—as you move your trunk forward. Eventually, you will be able to clasp your hands around your feet and rest your trunk and your forehead on your legs. Breathe normally and rhythmically as you hold this calm, restful position.

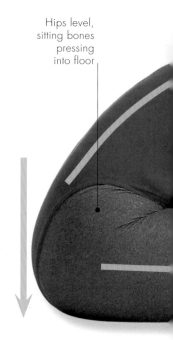

Hips level, sitting bones pressing into floor

Points to Watch

- Remember to breathe in before you stretch, and to reach forward on an out-breath.

- Keep your shoulders relaxed and your shoulder blades flat against your ribs.

- As you lean your trunk forward, imagine that your spine is straightening and lengthening.

Sitting forward bend analyzed

To achieve the full forward stretch in step 3 of the sitting forward bend on page 123, check the details pinpointed on the image below.

Legs together, kneecaps facing up, knees and ankles touching

Head relaxed, forehead resting on shins

Toes pointing up

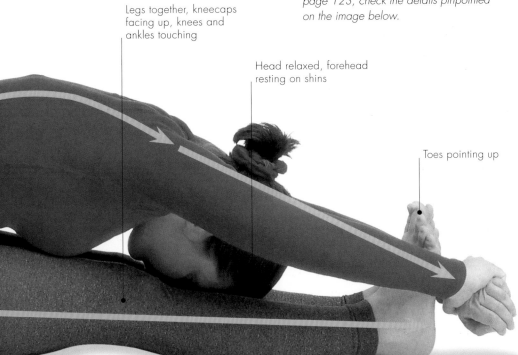

COBBLER FLOOR POSE

This lying-down version of the cobbler pose, **supta baddha konasana**, is a passive pose and a restful position. It provides a deep stretch across the groins, boosting the circulation to and from the pelvic area, and toning the muscles of the legs and hips.

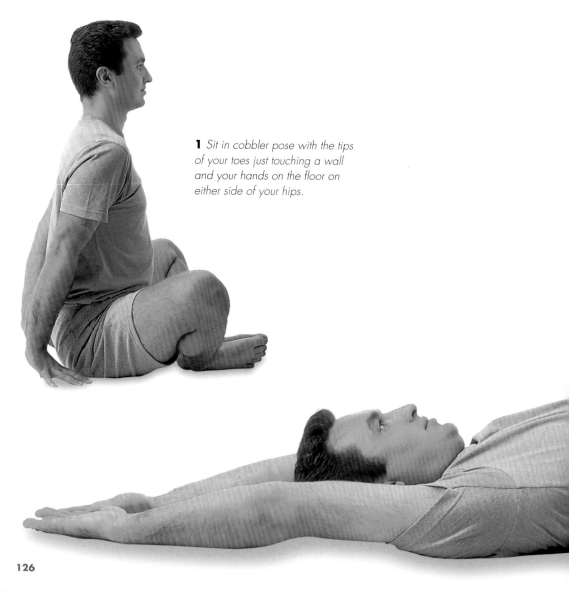

1 *Sit in cobbler pose with the tips of your toes just touching a wall and your hands on the floor on either side of your hips.*

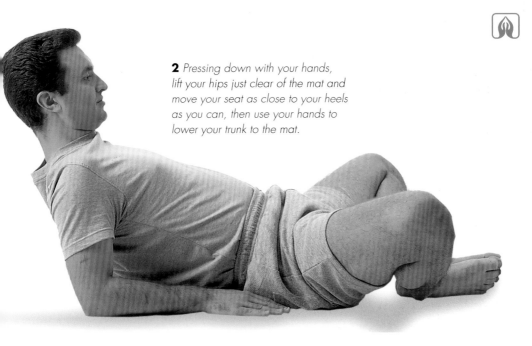

2 *Pressing down with your hands, lift your hips just clear of the mat and move your seat as close to your heels as you can, then use your hands to lower your trunk to the mat.*

3 *Raise your hips clear of the mat, move your seat closer to your heels, then lower your seat, rest your head on the mat, and relax your arms over your head. Hold this position for 1–2 minutes.*

Finish & rest

Place your arms on the mat by your sides, turn onto your side with your legs bent, then sit upright, straighten your legs, and rest.

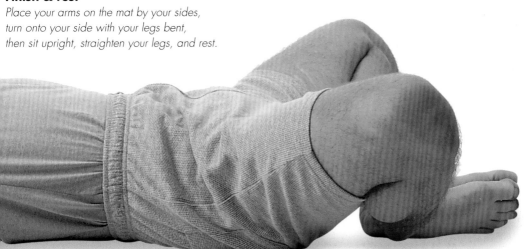

A Resting Pose

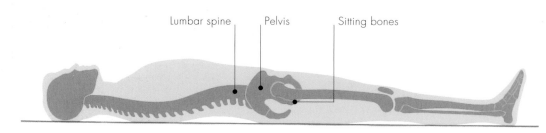

Lumbar spine   Pelvis   Sitting bones

I n some ways floor poses may seem harder work than standing poses, simply because a floor is hard, while the air gives readily. Looked at another way, however, floor poses are more restful than standing poses, because it is easier to relax when lying down. The cobbler floor pose is a perfect example. It is a passive pose—one in which you stretch, but do not change position—so it is more restful to perform lying on the floor than the sitting cobbler pose on page 110. But, like every lying-down pose, it will be restful only if the arch that forms in your

Avoiding strain
If you align your pelvis properly before lying back, your lumbar spine will be closer to the mat and more comfortable.

lower back when you lie down is reduced by stretching the lumbar spine. Lifting your hips and moving your seat toward your heels in step 2 is designed to achieve this.

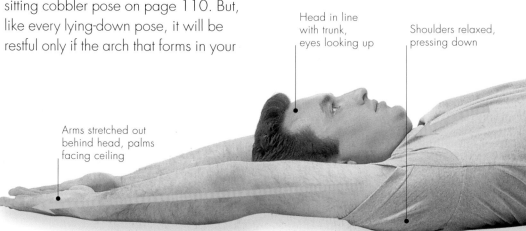

Head in line with trunk, eyes looking up

Shoulders relaxed, pressing down

Arms stretched out behind head, palms facing ceiling

Supporting the upper body

Before you start, place a blanket folded into a square on the floor between the points where your waist and head will be when you lie back, so that your upper back is supported. Your groins need to be as close as possible to your feet to get a good stretch across thighs and groins, but if your knees are stiff, leave more space between your groins and your feet. Lie squarely on the blanket and concentrate on stretching your lower back and your sitting bones away from your waist, toward the wall.

Points to Watch

- Start the pose with your toes touching a wall so that your feet do not creep steadily further away from your groins as you lie back and stretch.
- Keep your hip bones stretching toward your head and your sitting bones stretching toward your feet.

Cobbler floor pose analyzed

To achieve a good stretch in step 3 of the cobbler floor pose on page 127, check the details shown below.

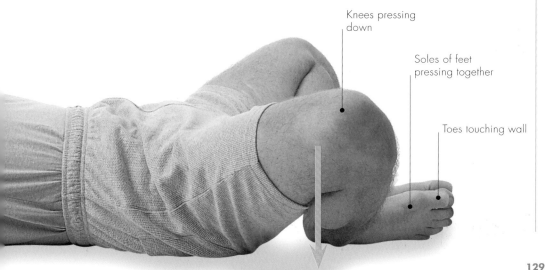

Knees pressing down

Soles of feet pressing together

Toes touching wall

DOWNWARD-FACING DOG This pose, called **adho mukha svanasana**, imitates a dog stretching with its rump in the air. It is a healing pose, capable of relieving stiffness in the shoulders and strain and tiredness in the legs and heels. It also relieves fatigue, since it slows the heartbeat and invigorates the brain and nervous system.

1 *Lie face down on a nonslip surface, with your elbows bent, your hands on the mat palms down, fingers spread out, fingertips just below your shoulders, your feet about 12 inches (30 centimeters) apart.*

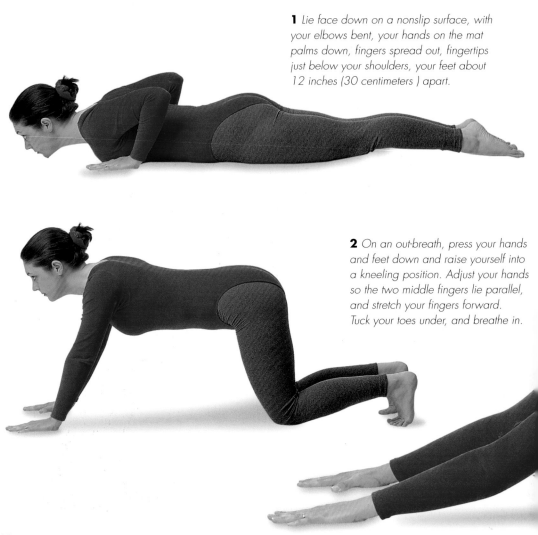

2 *On an out-breath, press your hands and feet down and raise yourself into a kneeling position. Adjust your hands so the two middle fingers lie parallel, and stretch your fingers forward. Tuck your toes under, and breathe in.*

Toes & Heels

Your feet remain 12 inches (30 centimeters) apart throughout the pose. In step 3, lower your heels as close to the floor as you comfortably can. Press them down to the mat as you stretch your legs up toward your hips.

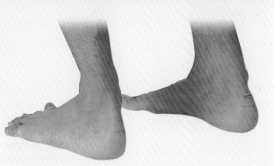

3 *Breathing out, lift your hips so your body forms an upside-down V-shape. Stretch your arms and trunk, and your legs, up toward your hips, pressing your hands and heels to the floor. Drop your head between your shoulders. Hold the stretch for 15–20 seconds.*

Finish & rest
Raise your head, bend your legs into a kneeling position, and rest in a kneeling forward bend.

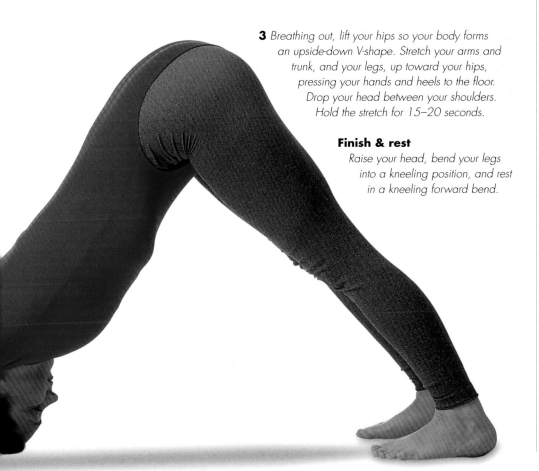

Gathering Energy

The downward-facing dog pose stretches the whole body, boosting the circulation, so it is an excellent antidote to fatigue. To achieve the full stretch, pay attention to the alignment of all parts of your body. Start by positioning your hands carefully, fingers spread out, middle fingers parallel, fingertips level with your shoulders. Start stretching from the moment you raise your hips. Press down on your feet and hands, and stretch your arms up, continuing the stretch along your sides.

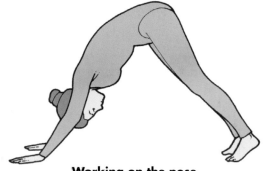

Working on the pose
If you can, check your reflection in a mirror to be sure that your body is making an inverted V. Your legs and back should be straighter than in the illustration above, and your heels lower. Stretch your trunk and legs up, away from your hands and feet.

Inverted V-shape

Your straight legs should form one side of an inverted V-shape, with your hips at the apex and your trunk and arms the other side. Do not walk your feet further forward to enable yourself to touch your heels to the floor while keeping your legs straight. The more you stretch up, the further down your heels will go, so instead, stretch up hard and work your heels further down. Press your feet into the floor, and stretch your thighs up to your hips at the apex of the V. At the same time, stretch your arms and trunk up toward your hips. Your neck is relaxed and your head

Arms straight, about 12 inches (30 centimeters) apart, and parallel

Hands flat on floor, fingers spread out, middle fingers aligned

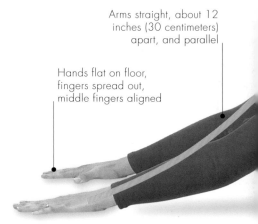

hangs, the crown touching the floor. Your feet, legs, and hands create a stretch all along the back of your body, while your abdomen remains relaxed.

Points to Watch

- Take care not to practice this pose on a rug or a slippery floor. Instead, practice on a mat with a nonslip undersurface, a wall-to-wall carpet, or other nonslip surface.

- Do not change the positions of your hands and feet while performing the pose. At the beginning of the pose you place your hands and feet in the right places for your body. If you move them, the pose will not be as effective.

Downward-facing dog pose analyzed

To achieve step 3 of the downward-facing dog pose on page 131, take time to assimilate all the details shown here.

Shoulders broad, shoulder blades flattened against ribs

Hips bones aligned

Legs straight, about 12 inches (30 centimeters) apart, and parallel

Heels touching floor

Crown of head touching floor

Toes tucked under shins, pointing to head

GATE POSE

In this pose, called **parighasana**, your body makes a shape rather like a gate with a crossbar formed by your trunk and outstretched arms. Like the triangle pose it stretches the sides of the body, but because you kneel and extend your trunk to the side, it is a little more demanding than the triangle.

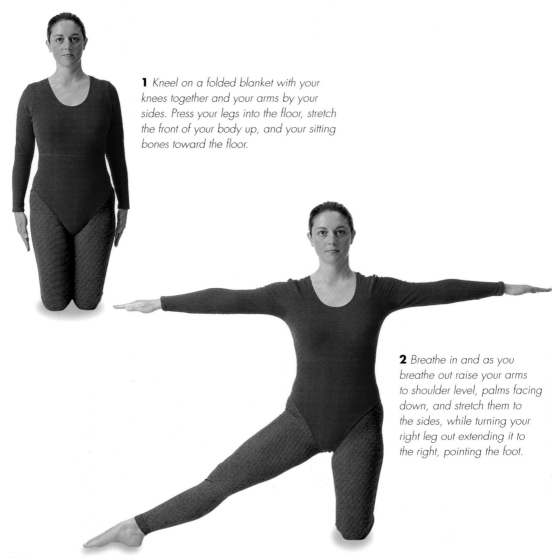

1 *Kneel on a folded blanket with your knees together and your arms by your sides. Press your legs into the floor, stretch the front of your body up, and your sitting bones toward the floor.*

2 *Breathe in and as you breathe out raise your arms to shoulder level, palms facing down, and stretch them to the sides, while turning your right leg out extending it to the right, pointing the foot.*

3 *Keeping your arms straight and your trunk facing directly forward, breathe in, and as you breathe out bend your trunk to the right from the hips until the back of your right hand touches your leg.*

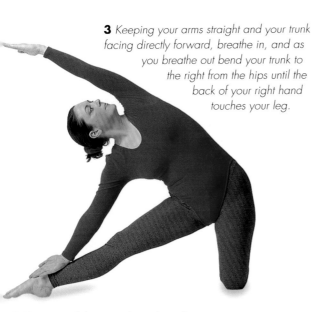

Raising Your Arm

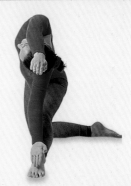

Keep your trunk facing forward and your shoulders level and broad so your upper arm lies along the side of your head. Work at stretching it back behind your ear.

4 *Move your left arm to the right until the upper arm lies over your left ear. Hold the stretch for up to 10 seconds.*

Repeat & finish
Repeat steps 1–4, bending to the left and stretching your left leg to the left. Return to step 1, sit back, and rest.

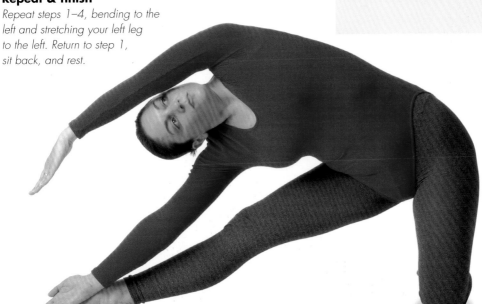

Sideways Extension

The gate pose is a sideways stretch that bends and extends the hips and abdomen in one movement, making it an excellent exercise for keeping the stomach and waist trim. Although this is a kneeling pose, stretching up at the beginning is the key to achieving the sideways extension, so pause in a kneeling position, press your legs firmly into the floor, and stretch from your knees all the way up the front of your body to the crown of your head, lifting your hip bones, and stretching your sitting bones down.

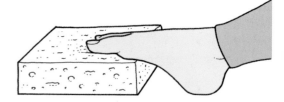

Working on the pose

If it is hard to rest the toes of your outstretched foot on the mat and keep your shin facing up, rest the foot on a foam block or a folded blanket.

Sideways extension

Be conscious of your shoulders as you raise your arms. Broaden across the collar bones while keeping your shoulder blades flattened against your ribs. As you bend your trunk, take care not to allow your shoulders and hips to roll forward. Instead, keep them in line, as if both buttocks and both shoulders were touching a wall. Keep your tailbone tucked in and your outstretched foot in line with your bent knee. Bend from the hips, keeping your trunk facing forward.

Extend your whole body from your hips as far to the side as you can, breathing normally and feeling the stretch from your thigh to your hip joint, and up both sides of your trunk.

Keep both arms straight, and bring them as close together above your head as you can. If at first you find it uncomfortable or difficult to narrow the gap between them, simply keep your upper arm vertical. As you practice, your hip and shoulder joints become more elastic, enabling you to bend further to the side until eventually the palms of your hands meet and the back of the lower hand rests on your foot.

- As you stretch your leg to one side, turn it out from the hip so your kneecap and shin bone face upward throughout the pose.

- As you bend your trunk to the right or the left, turn your face toward your upper arm and look up.

Gate pose analyzed

Stretching effectively in step 4 of the gate pose on page 135 depends on the details shown below. Note that your right shin and foot rest on the mat.

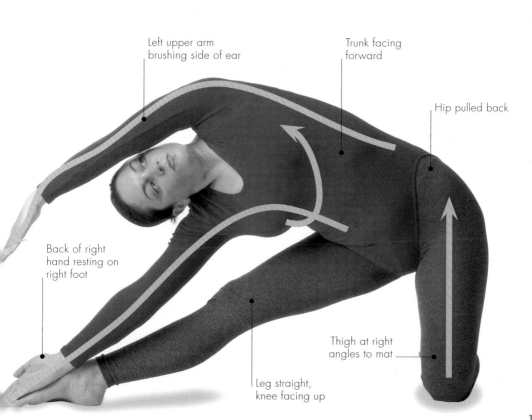

Left upper arm brushing side of ear

Trunk facing forward

Hip pulled back

Back of right hand resting on right foot

Thigh at right angles to mat

Leg straight, knee facing up

137

REVOLVING ABDOMEN

The ultimate posture for toning flabby abdominal muscles, **jathara parivartanasana** is an exercise that also improves the functioning of the liver, the spleen, the pancreas, and the intestines. It is said to be a good slimming exercise, and to relieve backache. The legs follow a half-circle as they swing from one side of the body to the other, giving the waist an invigorating stretch.

1 *Lie on your back on the mat, bend your legs, and stretch your arms out to the sides, palms facing up.*

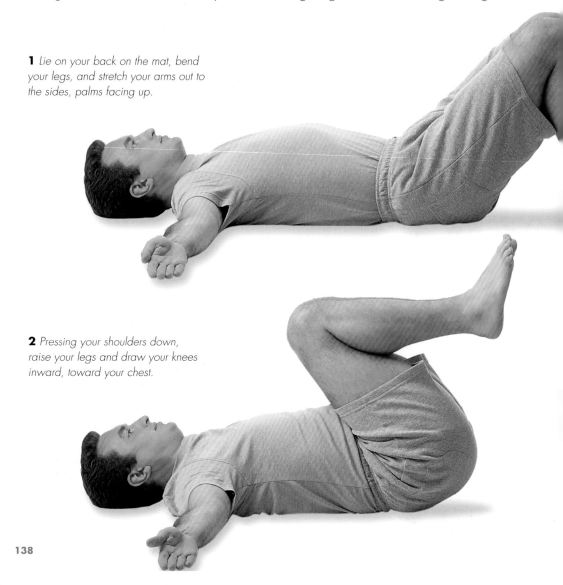

2 *Pressing your shoulders down, raise your legs and draw your knees inward, toward your chest.*

Aligning Your Shoulders

As you lower your knees to the right, do not lift your left shoulder. Both shoulders should remain aligned, touching the mat, through the pose.

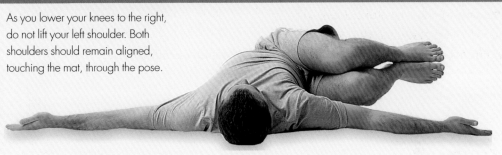

3 *Keeping your left shoulder on the mat, swing your knees over to the right while turning your abdomen (the part of the body between the diaphragm and pelvis) over to the left. Hold the position for 10–15 seconds.*

Repeat & finish
Raise your knees to your chest, then repeat step 3, this time swinging your knees over to the left and your abdomen to the right. Return to step 1, straighten your legs, and rest.

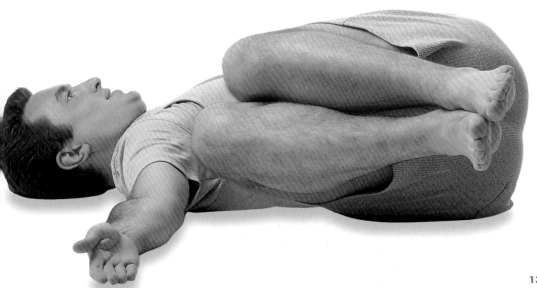

Massage Through Exercise

Swinging the legs slowly from side to side while keeping the upper back and shoulders on the floor twists the spine, and massages and stimulates the lower back, relieving backache. Raising the knees to the chest at the beginning of the pose stretches the lower back, so the spine can turn without strain. Raise your knees high up on your chest, then pause to extend your sitting bones away from your head, and to stretch from your hip bones to the top of your breastbone, and horizontally from your breastbone out to the fingertips of each hand.

Revolving the abdomen

Do not drop your legs to the floor, but lower them gently and deliberately on a slow out-breath, keeping your hips and trunk in line so as not to jar the spine. As you move your legs to the side, turn your abdomen in the opposite direction. If you keep your knees close to your chest and turn from the hips, this will stretch your back and waist.

Revolving abdomen analyzed
To achieve a massaging effect while moving your lower body right and left in the revolving abdomen pose on page 139, check the details shown here.

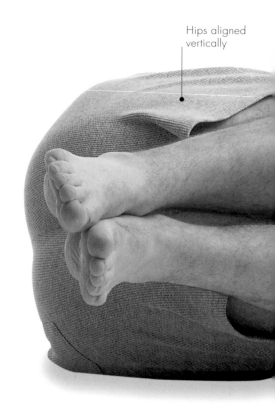

Hips aligned vertically

Points to Watch

- Keep your hips in vertical alignment throughout the pose. Do not allow the uppermost hip and the trunk to follow the movement of the legs and roll over.

- Keep both shoulders and as much of your back on the floor as you can when swinging your knees to right or left.

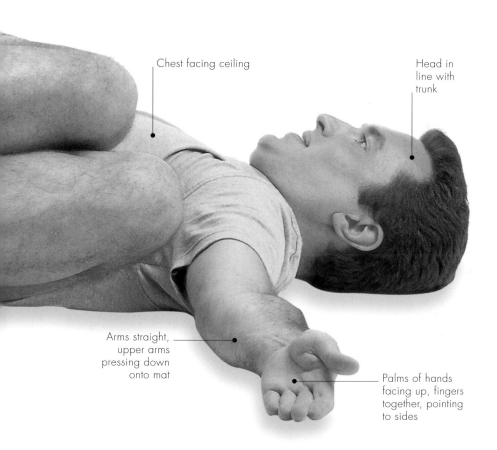

Chest facing ceiling

Head in line with trunk

Arms straight, upper arms pressing down onto mat

Palms of hands facing up, fingers together, pointing to sides

BOAT POSES

These two poses strengthen the muscles of the back and the stomach. Both are graded at the second level of difficulty, but half-boat, **ardha navasana**, demands more of the abdominal muscles than boat with oars, **paripurna navasana**. They vitalize the back and benefit the organs of digestion: the liver, gallbladder, spleen, and intestines.

Boat with oars

1 *Sit in the rod pose (see page 106), press your sitting bones down, and lift your spine and trunk. On an out-breath, incline your trunk back and raise your legs until your feet are higher than your head.*

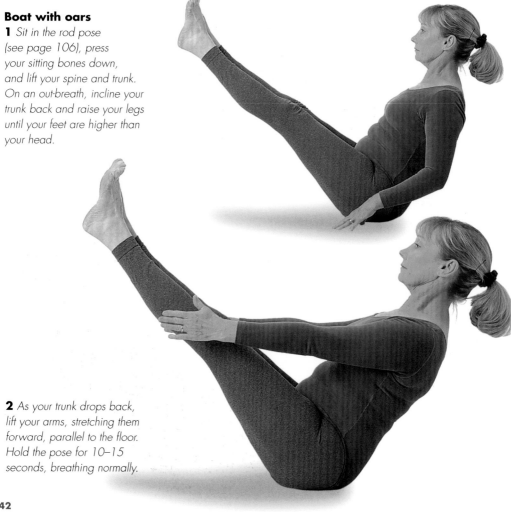

2 *As your trunk drops back, lift your arms, stretching them forward, parallel to the floor. Hold the pose for 10–15 seconds, breathing normally.*

Half-boat

1 *Sit in the rod pose, and clasp your hands behind your head, fingers interlocking, upper arms parallel and lifting. Press your sitting bones down to the floor, lift your spine, and raise your trunk.*

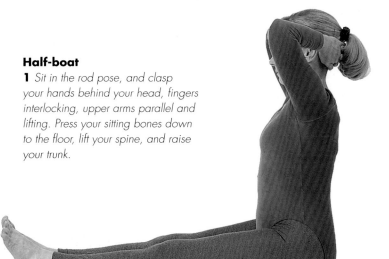

2 *Breathe in, and on the out-breath lower your trunk toward the floor and raise your legs until your toes are level with your eyes. Hold the pose for 5–10 seconds, then rest.*

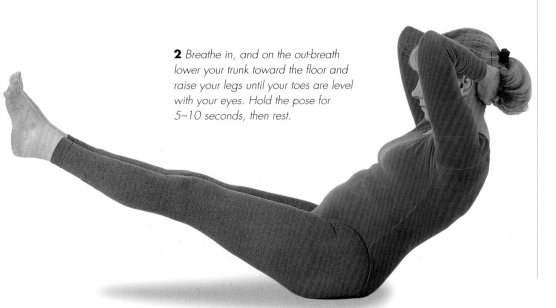

Maintaining Balance

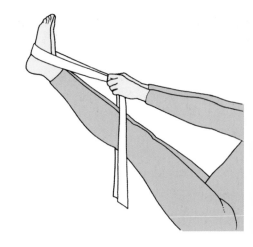

In the two boat poses on pages 142–43, you lower your back and raise your legs, so you balance on your buttocks. In boat with oars, the trunk and legs are raised at a 60° angle to the mat, so your body forms an almost perfect V-shape, but in the half-boat pose your back and legs are raised at a more oblique angle.

Keeping your balance

Stretching is the key to balancing in these poses: keep your spine and trunk lifting, press your sitting bones toward the floor, and keep your legs rod-straight, pressing together, and stretching toward your heels. Inhale as you stretch, exhale as you lift your legs and arms, then continue breathing normally to the end of the pose.

Rock back onto your sitting bones as you lift your legs. In boat with oars, place your hands on the floor beside your hips to balance until you have lifted your legs, then stretch your arms forward. If you find it hard to balance, bend your legs, clasp your hands around the backs of your knees, and pull on your legs, stretching your trunk up as you do so. Alternatively,

Boat with oars

If you find it difficult to hold the boat with oars pose, work on strengthening the muscles of your back and abdomen. One way is to loop a belt around your feet, hold an end in either hand, and pull on it, lifting and straightening your back.

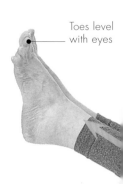

Toes level with eyes

place your feet against a wall to steady them, or rest your legs on a chair seat, holding the chair legs with your hands.

Points to Watch

- Do not hold your breath while holding the pose.

- If the muscles of your abdomen start to shake, ignore the shaking as long as there is no pain. It is a sign that the muscles are working.

- Keep your shoulders down and relaxed throughout, so your shoulder blades lie flat against your ribs. If tension mounts in your neck and shoulders, rest and work on the pose again later.

Half-boat pose analyzed

Sustaining your balance in the half-boat pose requires practice. Pay attention to each of the details shown here to help maintain the pose.

Head and neck upright, eyes looking forward

Upper arms lifting

Shoulders back, shoulder blades flattened against ribs

Trunk stretching up

Legs straight and stretching up at 30° angle

Lower back pressing in

FLOOR LEG-STRETCHES
The sequence of floor movements called **supta padangusthasana** stretches the legs and works the hips. Two movements are shown here. They boost the blood circulation in the lower body, so they are a good warming exercise for the legs and feet in cold weather. They also improve the flexibility of the hip joints.

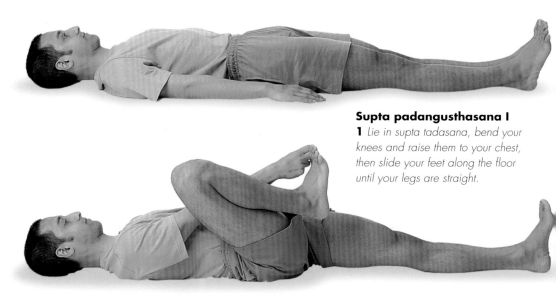

Supta padangusthasana I
1 *Lie in supta tadasana, bend your knees and raise them to your chest, then slide your feet along the floor until your legs are straight.*

2 *Press your left leg into the floor and lift your right leg, bending the knee to catch hold of the big toe with the fingers and thumb of your right hand.*

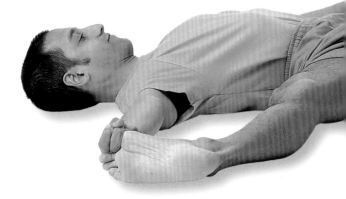

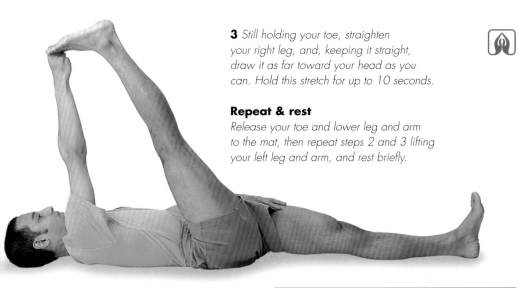

3 *Still holding your toe, straighten your right leg, and, keeping it straight, draw it as far toward your head as you can. Hold this stretch for up to 10 seconds.*

Repeat & rest

Release your toe and lower leg and arm to the mat, then repeat steps 2 and 3 lifting your left leg and arm, and rest briefly.

Holding the Toe

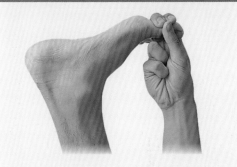

Hold your big toe between the thumb and index and middle fingers of your hand.

Supta padangusthasana II

4 *Repeat steps 1–3 of supta padangusthasana I, then put your left hand on your left thigh and press down hard, turn your right leg out from the hip, and lower your right leg and arm together to the floor. Hold this pose for up to 10 seconds.*

Repeat & finish

Rest in supta tadasana, then repeat step 4, grasping your left big toe with your left fingers and thumb, and lowering leg and arm to the left.

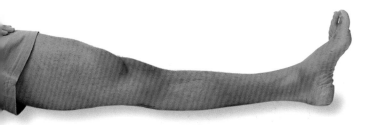

Working the Hip Joints

Keeping your legs straight through the leg-stretches on pages 146–47 will mobilize your hips and legs. At the beginning of each pose your knees, ankles, and big toes need to be touching, and when you raise one leg, do not disturb the alignment of the other. It remains pressing down on the mat and stretching toward the upturned toes through the remaining steps.

In step 3, stretch your right leg up and gradually draw it toward your head, feeling the stretch from hip to heel. Keep your foot at right angles to the leg, as it was when it left the floor. When you grasp your toe or pull on a belt, do not pull your toes down toward you, nor point them upward.

Second movement

The second movement in this sequence— padangusthasana II—is shown as step 4 on page 147. For this you need to turn your raised leg out a little at the hip joint before pulling it down to the floor to the right, pressing your left hip firmly down. Keep it straight and moving toward your head as you lower it, so that when it rests, your arm is in line with your shoulder.

Lower it just as far as you can at first. If necessary, rest it on foam yoga blocks by your trunk. In time you will be able to take it down to the floor.

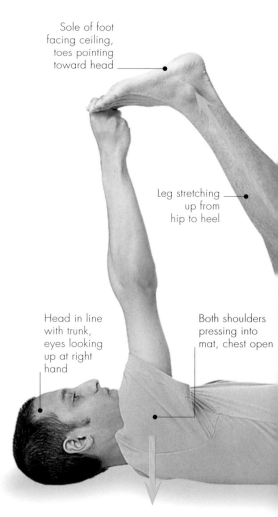

Sole of foot facing ceiling, toes pointing toward head

Leg stretching up from hip to heel

Head in line with trunk, eyes looking up at right hand

Both shoulders pressing into mat, chest open

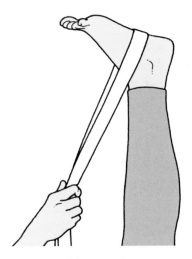

Working on the pose

If you cannot straighten your leg while holding your big toe, wind a belt around your foot in step 1 of padangusthasana I, and hold both ends in your raised hand, as close to your foot as you can.

Points to Watch

- Do lower your legs to the floor before straightening them in step 1. If you straighten them in the air, their weight will pull your pelvis up, arching your lower back. This can cause your back to strain.

- Do not let either leg roll out. Your knees, shin bones, and toes point directly up in steps 1 and 2, and the raised leg and foot point toward your head in step 3.

- If you use a belt in either pose, hold it in one hand while keeping your leg stretching up and your foot pressing into it.

Supta padangusthasana I analyzed

Follow the details shown in the diagram below to achieve step 3 of padangusthasana I on page 147.

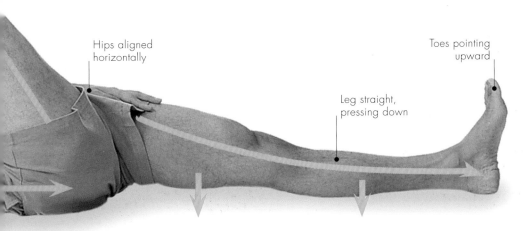

Hips aligned horizontally

Toes pointing upward

Leg straight, pressing down

HERO FLOOR POSE

Supta virasana is similar to hero pose shown on page 106, but performed lying on the floor with the arms extended over the head. This is a pose that stretches the entire front of the body, from the thighs to the neck, and it is a sure cure for leg ache for people who have to be on their feet all day.

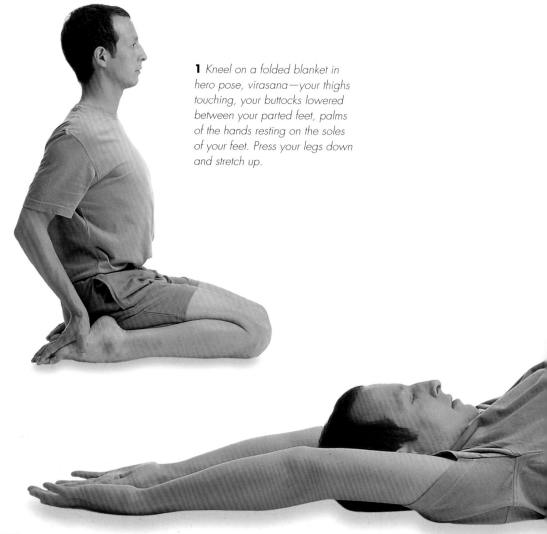

1 *Kneel on a folded blanket in hero pose, virasana—your thighs touching, your buttocks lowered between your parted feet, palms of the hands resting on the soles of your feet. Press your legs down and stretch up.*

2 *On an out-breath, bend back from the hips until your trunk rests on your elbows, your hands still holding the soles of your feet. Stretch your trunk toward your head and straighten your back by lifting your sitting bones off the floor, stretching them toward your feet, then lowering them.*

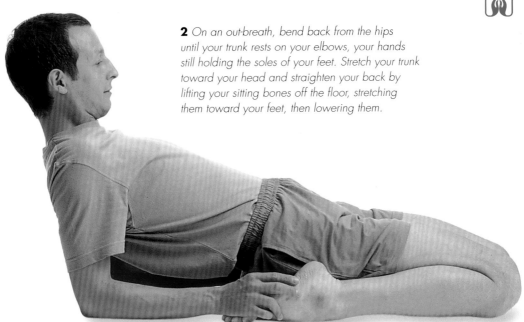

3 *Lower your back until your head rests on the mat. Release your hands, stretch your arms up and rest them, palms facing up, on the floor behind your head. Hold for 20 seconds or longer.*

Finish & rest
Lift your arms over your head and place your hands on your feet, raise your trunk onto your elbows as in step 2, sit up in hero pose, and rest.

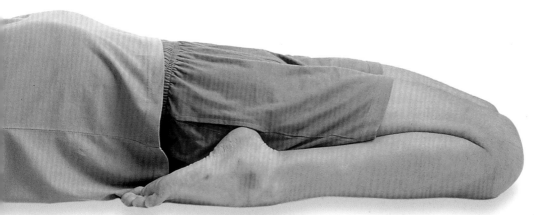

Relieving Aching Legs

Stretching any part of the body has an invigorating effect. We tend to stretch our upper body when we feel tired. This pose is effective for aching legs because it stretches the lower body—the thighs, knees, ankles, and feet, as well as the abdomen and trunk—resting muscles and improving circulation within the whole area.

Before moving back onto your elbows, stretch your spine from your pelvis to the crown of your head, press your sitting bones down, and level your hips. Lifting your buttocks just clear of the floor

stretching your sitting bones toward your knees in step 2 prevents strain when you lie back, so continue stretching as you lie, pulling up from your hips. Keep your thighs touching, but when you stretch your arms back over your head, rest your hands on the floor about 12 inches (30 centimeters) apart. Relax your abdomen. Do not push it out or up.

Using supports

If your seat does not reach the mat when you kneel in virasana in step 1, place one or two folded blankets behind you, so when

Hero floor pose analyzed

This illustration pinpoints the many details to think about in step 3 of the hero floor pose on page 151.

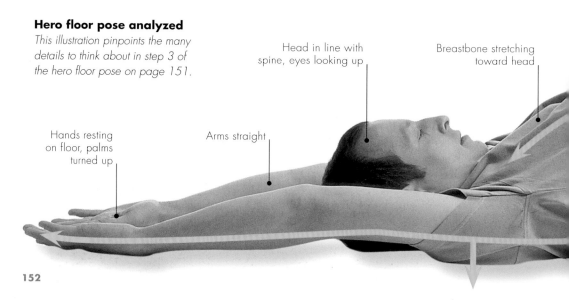

Head in line with spine, eyes looking up

Breastbone stretching toward head

Hands resting on floor, palms turned up

Arms straight

you lie back your upper body rests on them. If your knees are stiff, kneel on a blanket; and if you find you resist dropping back onto the floor, accustom yourself by lowering your back onto a pile of cushions or a row of foam blocks placed so that they support you from just above your waist up to your head.

Points to Watch

- Stretch upward from the groins to the fingertips and downward from the sitting bones to the knees.

- Keep the tops of your thighs facing up. Do not let them roll in toward each other.

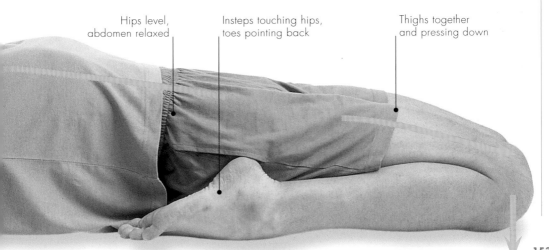

Hips level, abdomen relaxed

Insteps touching hips, toes pointing back

Thighs together and pressing down

FOUR-LIMBED POSES
The four-limbed rod or **chaturanga dandasana** is a strengthening exercise, the Eastern version of press-ups, with the difference that you push up once, then hold. In contrast, the side-reclining leg lift pose, **anantasana**, is a reclining pose. It relieves back strain and tones the pelvic area.

Side-reclining leg lift pose
1 *Lie on your mat on your left side, with your legs straight and stretching toward your feet, your right arm along your right side, palm resting on your thigh.*

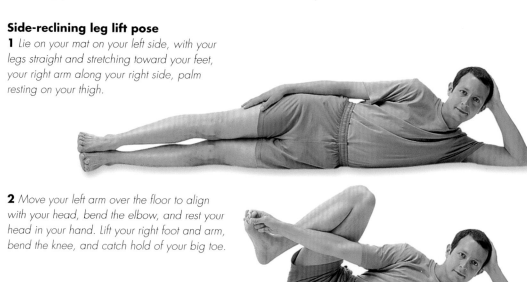

2 *Move your left arm over the floor to align with your head, bend the elbow, and rest your head in your hand. Lift your right foot and arm, bend the knee, and catch hold of your big toe.*

3 *Now straighten the leg and move it back in line with your trunk. Hold for up to 20 seconds.*

Repeat & finish
Bend your knee and lower your leg, letting go of your toe and dropping your arm to the floor, and rest briefly in supta tadasana. Repeat steps 1–3, lying on your right side and lifting your left leg.

Four-limbed rod pose

1 *Lie face down with your feet about 12 inches (30 centimeters) apart, your heels raised, your elbows bent, and your hands palms down on the floor beside your chest. Spread your fingers, move your elbows toward each other, and stretch them toward your feet.*

2 *Raise your head and look forward. Breathe in, stretch your legs toward your heels and your breastbone toward your head and press your toes and hands down. Breathe out, and lift your thighs and trunk to align with your heels. Hold for up to 10 seconds, breathing normally. On an out-breath, lower your trunk to the floor, turn onto your back, and lie with your knees bent.*

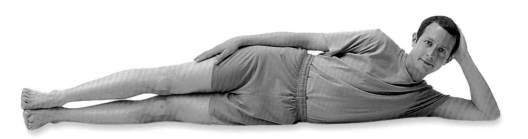

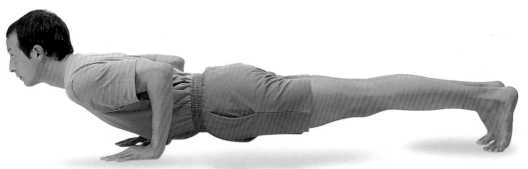

Using the Floor

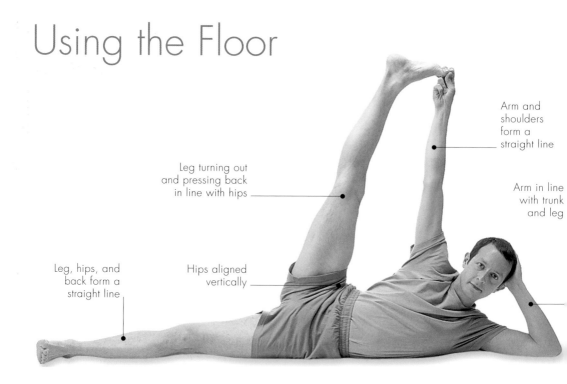

Arm and shoulders form a straight line

Arm in line with trunk and leg

Leg turning out and pressing back in line with hips

Leg, hips, and back form a straight line

Hips aligned vertically

Anantasana, the Sanskrit name for the side-reclining leg lift pose on page 154, is the name of the serpent whose coils formed the couch on which reclined the Hindu god, Vishnu, and it is a fundamentally restful pose. It demands attention to alignment, so begin by checking that your ankles, legs, trunk, and shoulders are in line. Keep your sitting bones stretching toward your feet, your hip bones lifting toward your head, and your tailbone pressing in. Your raised leg should be pressed back in line with your hips.

Side-reclining leg lift pose analyzed

The image above analyzes step 3 of the side-reclining leg lift pose on page 154. To perfect the pose, check the details in your reflection in a mirror.

If you find you cannot straighten your leg while holding your toe, do not pull it forward. Instead, wind a belt around your foot and hold the two ends as you lift your leg vertically above your hips, pressing your foot into the belt. Finally, do not allow the upper side of your trunk to roll forward. Shoulders and trunk should align vertically.

Pressing up

The four-limbed rod pose strengthens the wrists and the muscles of the shoulders, arms, and abdomen. You need to make your legs as stiff as a rod or staff, so before lifting, tighten the muscles at the sides of your thighs, press your tailbone in, and stretch from hips to breastbone. Press your hands and feet down to the floor to raise your trunk and legs. If you find this difficult, lie with the soles of your feet against a wall and press them into it. Use this technique if you find it hard to balance in the side-reclining leg lift pose.

Four-limbed rod pose analyzed

If you find it hard to lift from the floor in step 2 of the four-limbed rod pose on page 155, check each of the details shown here. Placing each hand on a foam yoga block also helps you lift.

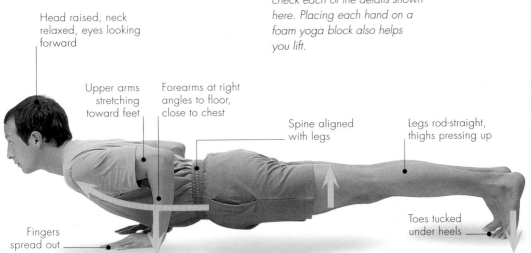

Head raised, neck relaxed, eyes looking forward

Upper arms stretching toward feet

Forearms at right angles to floor, close to chest

Spine aligned with legs

Legs rod-straight, thighs pressing up

Fingers spread out

Toes tucked under heels

CROSS-LEGGED TWIST

Here, the cross-legged sitting pose or **sukhasana** is transformed into a twist: sitting upright and keeping the spine stretching up, you rotate it right and then left. Not only does this pose make the spine more flexible but it also feels good. Before attempting the exercises on pages 158–92, please read carefully the caution note on page 9.

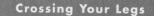

Crossing Your Legs

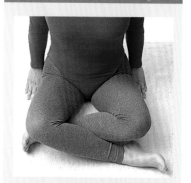

Do not cross your legs too tightly or you will pull your spine out of its natural alignment and you will not be able to stretch it up. There should be a sizeable gap between your calves and your groins.

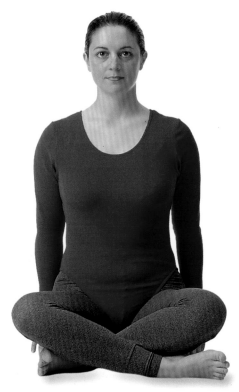

1 *Sit in the rod pose (see page 106) and cross your right leg over your left leg as shown on page 38. Place your hands on the mat beside your hips, and stretch your spine up.*

Working on the Pose

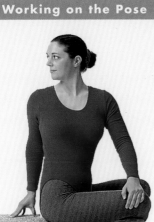

Sit on a foam block or a blanket folded two or three times, and place another close behind you. Pressing your hand onto it while you turn keeps your spine upright. To twist further, walk your hand as far around as you can.

2 *Turn your trunk to the right and place your left hand on the outside of your right leg and your right hand close behind you. Press that hand down and pull with your left hand to rotate further. Look over your right shoulder and twist for 10–15 seconds.*

Repeat & finish

Return to step 1, then repeat step 2, this time crossing your left leg over your right and twisting to the left. Rest, and repeat the pose.

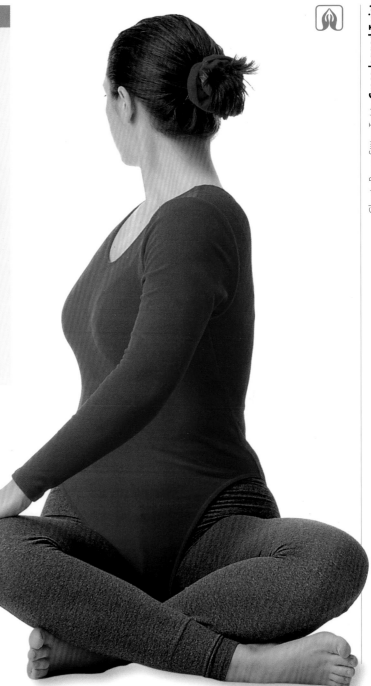

Introducing Sitting Twists

Many a back problem starts with an abrupt turn to reach something behind the back. If the muscles that rotate the spine are well exercised they respond easily to a sudden turn, but if they are tight through lack of exercise an awkward movement can strain them. The next few pages concentrate on the twists, which gently exercise the many small muscles that rotate the spine. The standing chair twist on page 74 introduced the twists; the three twists in this chapter are performed sitting down.

Helping your spine turn

A twist will only be effective if your back is straight when you rotate it. Sitting on a foam block or a blanket folded two or three times will help you lift your back. When you sit down, roll or pull the large buttock muscles out to the sides. Then with your trunk facing forward and your legs pressing down, stretch your spine up. Use your hands to help yourself turn. The hand pressing down behind you keeps you upright, and pulling on your knee with the other twists you further around. Never let your spine collapse—keep it stretching up, even when you turn to the front.

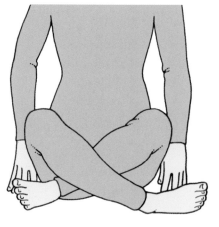

Positioning the knees

When you cross your legs, your knees should lie close to the floor. If you find it difficult to lower them, cross them at the shins, then move them toward each other before pressing them down.

Points to Watch

- Lift and open your upper chest, pressing your shoulders down and back.

- As you turn, level your shoulders so that one side of your chest does not rise higher than the other side.

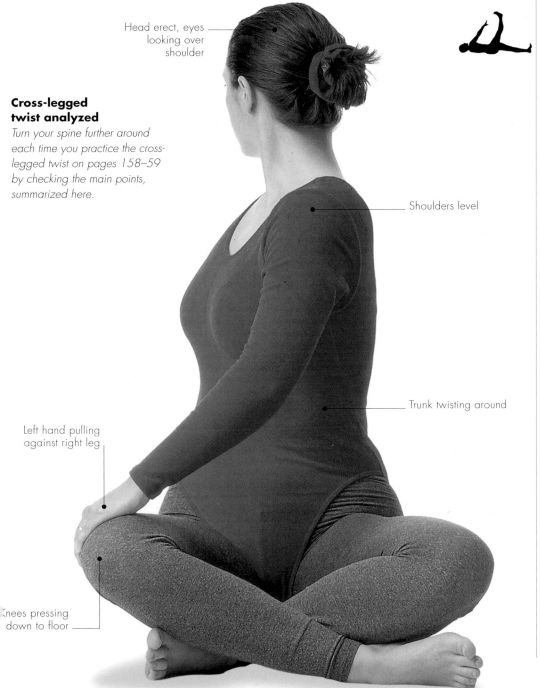

Head erect, eyes looking over shoulder

Cross-legged twist analyzed

Turn your spine further around each time you practice the cross-legged twist on pages 158–59 by checking the main points, summarized here.

Shoulders level

Trunk twisting around

Left hand pulling against right leg

Knees pressing down to floor

MERMAID I

In this pose your legs, bent to the side of you, look like a mermaid's tail. But its Sanskrit name, Bharadvajasana, commemorates the warrior Bharadvaja, a mythical figure from the Hindu epic, *Mahabharata*. This pose, **Bharadvajasana I**, rotates the spine, exercising the middle and upper spine particularly, dispelling stiffness and making your back feel supple.

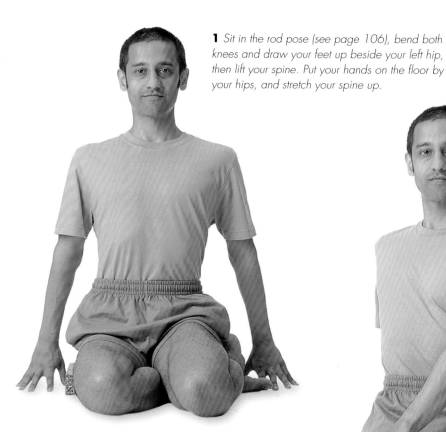

1 *Sit in the rod pose (see page 106), bend both knees and draw your feet up beside your left hip, then lift your spine. Put your hands on the floor by your hips, and stretch your spine up.*

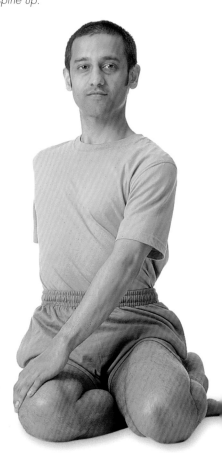

2 *Breathing out, turn your trunk from the hips to the right. Place your left hand on your right thigh and pull gently to rotate to the right, and press your right hand down behind you to lift and rotate further.*

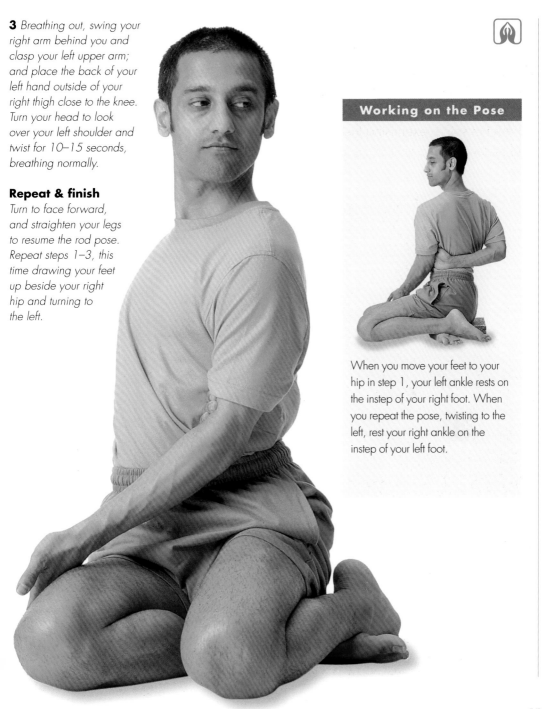

3 *Breathing out, swing your right arm behind you and clasp your left upper arm; and place the back of your left hand outside of your right thigh close to the knee. Turn your head to look over your left shoulder and twist for 10–15 seconds, breathing normally.*

Repeat & finish

Turn to face forward, and straighten your legs to resume the rod pose. Repeat steps 1–3, this time drawing your feet up beside your right hip and turning to the left.

Working on the Pose

When you move your feet to your hip in step 1, your left ankle rests on the instep of your right foot. When you repeat the pose, twisting to the left, rest your right ankle on the instep of your left foot.

Spiraling

To be effective, twists need to be performed as gently and precisely as any other movement in yoga. The idea is to rotate the spine as far as it will comfortably go, not to wrench it around. Rotation takes place mainly in the upper back—the thoracic area of the spine (see pages 26–27). Here, the joints between the 12 thoracic vertebrae, the ligaments that bind them, and the muscles that move them respond to stretching and exercise. If you practice this twist regularly and gently, you find that your spine will twist a little further around each time.

Learning to spiral

From the beginning of step 1, every movement in the mermaid pose contributes to helping the spine spiral. You start by sitting in the rod pose and lifting your whole trunk from the hips. Lifting your trunk strengthens the upward stretch, making it easier to turn the trunk from the hips. Start turning on an out-breath, and keep up the momentum by stretching your sitting bones down, and pressing one hand firmly down and the other against your thigh to rotate your body further right or left. Finally, the

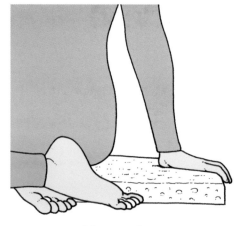

Working on the pose
Press your hand down into a foam block or a blanket folded two or three times and placed behind you. This helps you lever your trunk further around during the twist.

actions of swinging one hand behind your back to clasp the other arm, and turning your head to look over your shoulder, cause your body to spiral just that little further. Holding the pose for a few seconds, still stretching up, accustoms your trunk to turning, making the pose easier next time.

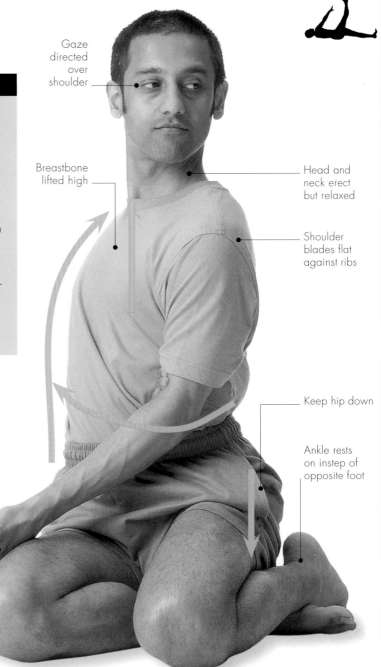

Points to Watch

- Do not disturb the balance of your hips when you move your feet, or when you turn. Keep both sitting bones pressing down and your hip bones level. If this is difficult, raise your pelvis on two folded blankets or on a foam block with a folded blanket laid on top.

- Keep your shoulders in line— do not allow one to rise higher than the other when you twist your trunk.

Mermaid 1 analyzed

Check the details shown in the illustration on the right to achieve a good twist in step 3 of the mermaid 1 pose shown on page 163.

Back of hand resting beneath thigh, close to knee

Knees touching floor, facing forward

Gaze directed over shoulder

Breastbone lifted high

Head and neck erect but relaxed

Shoulder blades flat against ribs

Keep hip down

Ankle rests on instep of opposite foot

165

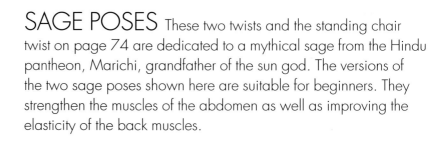

SAGE POSES
These two twists and the standing chair twist on page 74 are dedicated to a mythical sage from the Hindu pantheon, Marichi, grandfather of the sun god. The versions of the two sage poses shown here are suitable for beginners. They strengthen the muscles of the abdomen as well as improving the elasticity of the back muscles.

Marichyasana I

1 *Sit in the rod pose (see page 106) on a foam block or a folded blanket, bend your left knee, drawing your heel toward your left buttock, then grasp your shin with both hands and pull your trunk forward toward your thigh.*

2 *Press your right hand down behind you and lift from the hips. Bend your left arm, stretch it forward, and press the elbow against the inside of your bent knee. Then press your right leg and right hand down, lift your trunk, and twist to the right.*

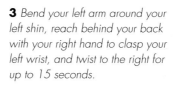

3 *Bend your left arm around your left shin, reach behind your back with your right hand to clasp your left wrist, and twist to the right for up to 15 seconds.*

Repeat & finish
Return to rod pose and repeat steps 1 and 2, bending your right leg, pressing your right elbow against your right knee, and turning left.

Marichyasana III

1 *Sit in the rod pose, bend your right knee, draw the heel toward the buttock, clasp the bent knee with your hands, and pull your trunk toward it. Pressing your left leg down, lift from the hips and keeping your spine stretching forward and up, pull on your shin.*

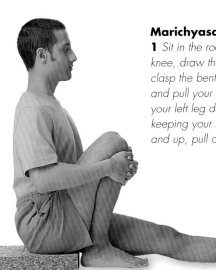

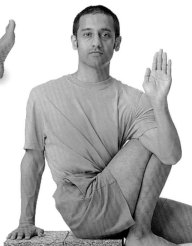

2 *Press your right hand on the floor behind you to assist the lift and turning from the hips, rotate your trunk to the right. Pressing your left elbow against the outside of the knee, use it to lever your trunk further to the right.*

3 *Bend your left arm around your right shin, reach behind your back with your right hand to clasp your left wrist. Hold for 15 seconds.*

Repeat & finish

Return to the rod pose, then repeat steps 1–3, bending your left leg, pressing your right elbow against the outside of your left knee, and twisting to the left.

˙Powered Rotation

These two poses use the elbow as a powerful lever to rotate the spine from the hips more strongly. They give the trunk an intense stretch, which increases the blood supply to the kidneys. It is essential to stretch the trunk strongly upward before turning the spine, and to propel it forward to keep it perpendicular to the floor. To do this, you clasp the shin of your bent leg with your hands, just below the knee, and pull on it, drawing your trunk toward your upstretched thigh.

Keep your spine lifting by pressing down into the floor with your outstretched leg and press one hand onto the floor or on a foam yoga block placed behind you.

Using leverage
Bringing the elbow against your bent knee in step 2 of both twists enables you to use it as a lever to turn your trunk. To do this effectively, keep the knee upright, and pull your trunk forward. There should be no space between your armpit and the top of your thigh where it rests. Breathe in before you place your elbow against your knee, and as you exhale, stretch your trunk forward and upward, and press

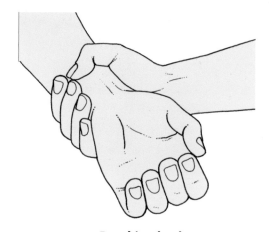

Reaching back
Reach behind your back in step 3 of both poses to grasp the wrist of the opposite arm firmly between your thumb and fingers.

elbow against knee and knee against elbow to rotate still more. Involve your whole trunk in the turn, revolving your abdomen, your waist, your chest, and your head in the direction of the twist.

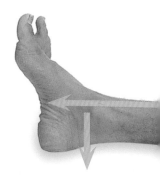

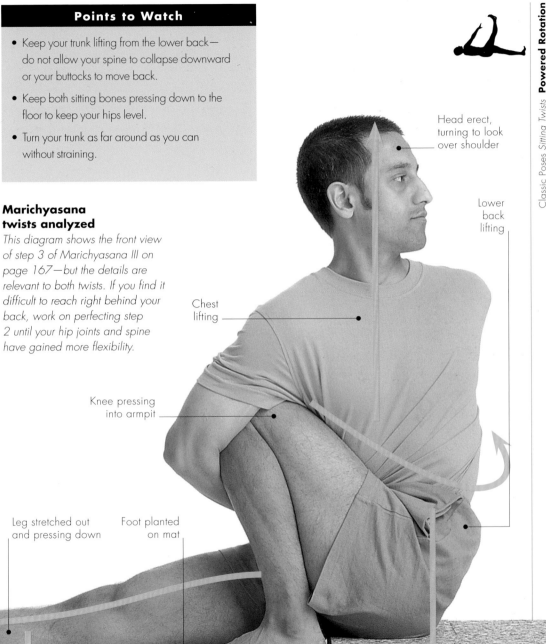

Points to Watch

- Keep your trunk lifting from the lower back—do not allow your spine to collapse downward or your buttocks to move back.

- Keep both sitting bones pressing down to the floor to keep your hips level.

- Turn your trunk as far around as you can without straining.

Marichyasana twists analyzed

This diagram shows the front view of step 3 of Marichyasana III on page 167—but the details are relevant to both twists. If you find it difficult to reach right behind your back, work on perfecting step 2 until your hip joints and spine have gained more flexibility.

Head erect, turning to look over shoulder

Lower back lifting

Chest lifting

Knee pressing into armpit

Leg stretched out and pressing down

Foot planted on mat

BRIDGE

The name of this pose, **sarvangasana setu bandha**, describes the bridge shape you make with your body by raising your back, using your shoulders and feet as supports. This is a good movement to follow a shoulder stand, since it gives the back a very remedial stretch.

1 *Lie on your back on the mat, your feet a hip-width apart and your arms by your sides. Bending your knees, move your heels toward your groins and stretch your sitting bones toward your heels.*

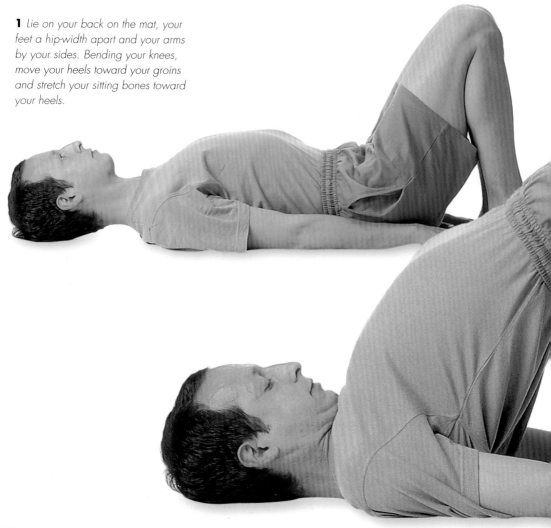

In order to give your spine even more of a stretch and to open your chest, raise the hips higher by lifting on to the balls of your feet. Then, as you retain the lift, lower your heels to the floor.

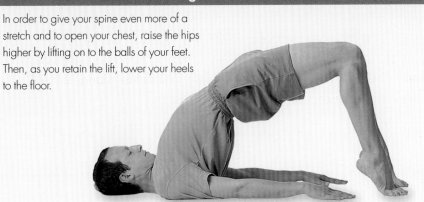

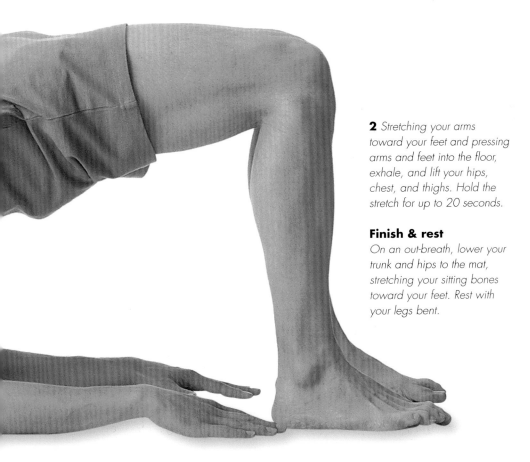

2 *Stretching your arms toward your feet and pressing arms and feet into the floor, exhale, and lift your hips, chest, and thighs. Hold the stretch for up to 20 seconds.*

Finish & rest

On an out-breath, lower your trunk and hips to the mat, stretching your sitting bones toward your feet. Rest with your legs bent.

Bending the Back

To retain its full mobility, the spine needs to be flexed backward, as well as forward and to the sides, and this section of Chapter 4 focuses on backbends performed while lying and kneeling. The bridge, which begins the sequence, involves actively lifting the back off of the floor. Begin in a good supta tadasana (see page 39), bending the legs before lifting, and stretching the sitting bones down toward the feet.

Making the bridge

To lift, press your arms hard into the floor, and raise your hips, using the large muscles of your buttocks and thighs and the many muscles that control the movements of the spine. As you rise, press your feet down hard on the mat, and stretch upward from the backs of your thighs. In order to arch the back high above the mat, raise your heels, lift your hips still higher, then lower your heels, keeping your hips lifting.

At first you may be able to raise your back just a little way, and to sustain the lift for a few seconds only. However, regular practice strengthens the muscles you use to lift your body, making your back more supple. Eventually, you may

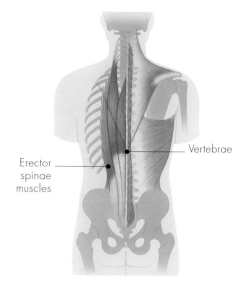

Erector spinae muscles

Vertebrae

Muscles that move the spine

Many small muscles, each attached to two or three vertebrae, work together to bend the spine back, forward, to either side, and to rotate it. They are called the erector spinae because they also hold the spine upright.

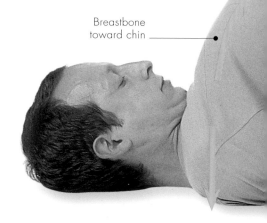

Breastbone toward chin

attempt a more advanced form of the pose—dropping the legs and feet down into the bridge from the shoulder stand, salamba sarvangasana, on pages 186–87.

Points to Watch

- To increase the lift, stretch your breastbone toward your head, and open your shoulders, pressing your shoulder blades against your ribs.

- Keep your chest, hips, tailbone, and thighs lifting throughout the pose.

- Relax your neck and your chin.

Bridge pose analyzed
Work through each detail shown here to maximize lift in the bridge pose on page 171.

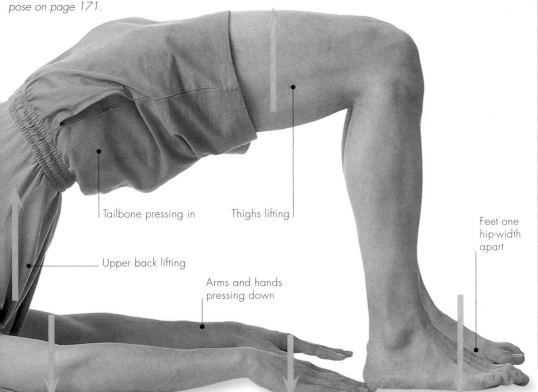

Tailbone pressing in

Thighs lifting

Feet one hip-width apart

Upper back lifting

Arms and hands pressing down

LOCUST

The name of this pose is descriptive—your body imitates the shape of a locust at rest. Authorities recommend the locust pose or **salabhasana** as a gentle exercise for strengthening the muscles around any part of the spine where a disk has slipped, and it certainly relieves backaches. It is more effective than sit-ups for exercising the large muscles of the abdomen, buttocks, and thighs.

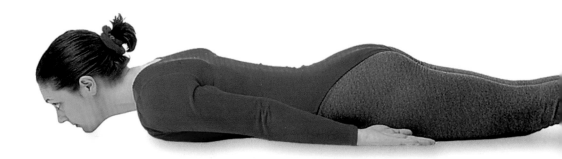

1 Lie on your stomach with your chin resting on the mat, your eyes facing the floor, your arms by your sides and legs together, both stretching back, and your palms turned up.

2 Press your pelvis into the floor, inhale, and, stretching your arms and hands toward your heels, lift your head, upper body, and legs as high off the floor as you can. Stretch your arms and legs back, level with your shoulders.

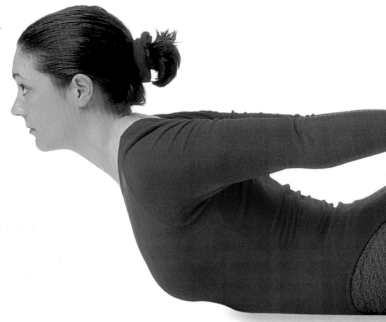

Legs & Feet

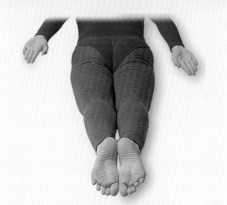

Keep your legs and feet together and your shins pointing directly downward—do not let your legs roll outward. Stretch your legs and feet away from your head. If at first you get a cramp when you stretch your feet back, stop and resume the pose when it has passed. It happens when muscles are unused to being stretched, so keep practicing and the cramps will disappear.

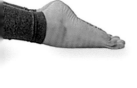

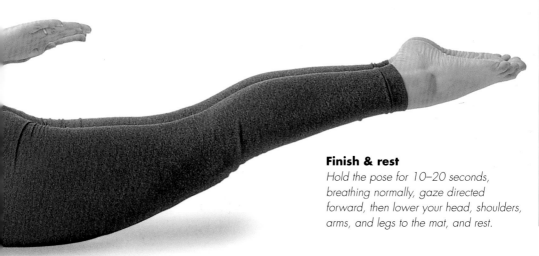

Finish & rest

Hold the pose for 10–20 seconds, breathing normally, gaze directed forward, then lower your head, shoulders, arms, and legs to the mat, and rest.

175

Arching the Back

From the neck down to the pelvis, each pair of vertebrae that form the spine is separated by a joint capable of just a small amount of movement. These partly movable joints, as they are called, all work together to give the spine its marvelous mobility. To remain fully mobile, however, the spine needs to be exercised regularly. In the course of a normal day we may occasionally bend forward to pick something up, twist around, and perhaps bend to one side or the other, but we rarely, if ever, bend the spine back.

Creating the arch

In the locust pose on pages 174–75 you bend the back while lying on your stomach, lifting your legs and thighs and your chest and shoulders off the mat, so that you balance on your lower abdomen and hip bones.

Arching the spine helps restore suppleness to the lower back especially, reducing discomfort in that often painful area. Strengthening the muscles that control the movements of the spine prevents disks from slipping. Arching also stimulates the digestive system, relieving indigestion and stomachache.

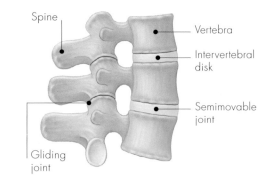

Spine

Vertebra

Intervertebral disk

Semimovable joint

Gliding joint

Joints of the spine

Disks of cartilage cushion the joints between vertebrae, allowing a little movement back, forward, and to the sides. When the vertebrae move, their spines glide over each other.

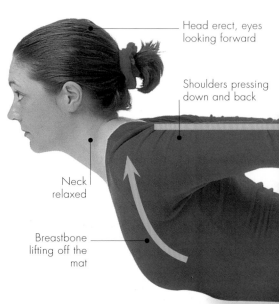

Head erect, eyes looking forward

Shoulders pressing down and back

Neck relaxed

Breastbone lifting off the mat

As you lift, you really stretch both arms and legs back, away from your head, and the trunk forward, toward it, so practicing this pose strengthens the abdominal muscles that lift the front of the body. The stronger these muscles become, the easier the pose will be.

Points to Watch

• Breathe in as you lift your chest and legs, then remember to breathe normally as you hold the pose.

• As you lift your legs and arms, really stretch them back, away from your head, and keep stretching throughout.

• Lift your breastbone as high as you can, but flatten your shoulder blades into your back.

Locust pose analyzed
The details shown here help you achieve lift in step 2 of the locust pose on page 175.

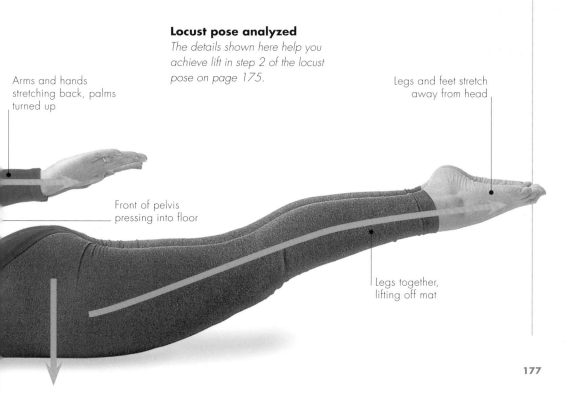

Arms and hands stretching back, palms turned up

Legs and feet stretch away from head

Front of pelvis pressing into floor

Legs together, lifting off mat

CAMEL

Ustrasana or camel pose intensifies the backward stretch of the spine, yet it is not too demanding, even if your back is stiff. It is an excellent pose for correcting poor posture—the rounded shoulders and back that result from too much sitting and slumping.

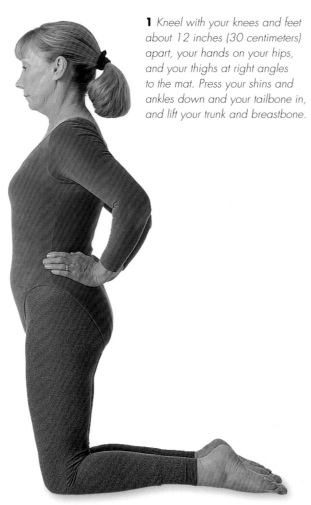

1 *Kneel with your knees and feet about 12 inches (30 centimeters) apart, your hands on your hips, and your thighs at right angles to the mat. Press your shins and ankles down and your tailbone in, and lift your trunk and breastbone.*

Working Behind the Back

If you have trouble guiding your hands to your feet with your arms behind you, hold a belt between finger and thumb of each hand, leaving 12 inches (30 centimeters) between them. Your hands are now the same distance apart as your heels, palms turned forward, so the belt will guide your hands down to your feet.

2 *Breathe out, drop your head back, take your arms behind your back, and place the palms of your hands on your feet, fingers pointing down. Lift from your thighs, stretching your breastbone up. Hold the stretch for up to 15 seconds.*

Finish & rest

Breathe in, lift your hands, and raise your head and trunk until you are kneeling upright. Relax, sitting on your heels with your hands on your thighs.

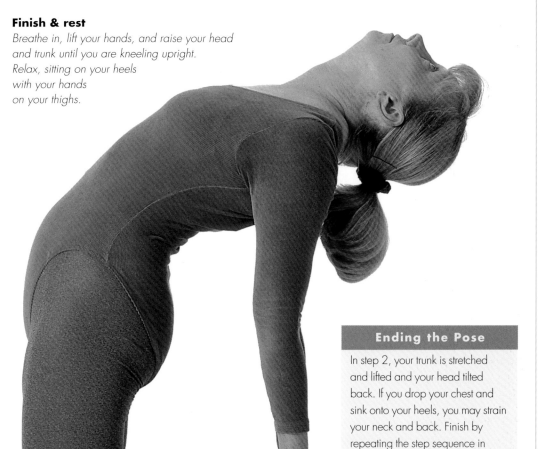

Ending the Pose

In step 2, your trunk is stretched and lifted and your head tilted back. If you drop your chest and sink onto your heels, you may strain your neck and back. Finish by repeating the step sequence in reverse, rather than just stopping midpose. Keep your spine stretching up.

179

Stretching the Trunk

The camel pose is more than a backbend since it stretches the whole of the trunk from the thighs to the neck. As you press your legs into the floor in step 1, you pull your tailbone in and stretch your sitting bones down toward the floor, and you lift your thighs and pull your trunk up from the groins and the hips to the top of the breastbone. As you move your hands back toward your heels, you stretch your shoulders back so your shoulder blades lie flat against your ribs, and the stretch runs along your arms to your hands. Keep both sides of the trunk in line so both hands reach the feet at the same time.

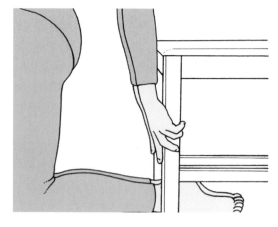

Overcoming resistance
To accustom yourself to bending your trunk back, place a chair behind you with its back against a wall, and bend backward, holding the chair legs with your hands.

Bending back

People sometimes find it difficult to bend their head and trunk back. When you first practice the pose, you may prefer to keep your head upright throughout the exercise until you feel comfortable enough to try bending back a little more each time you practice. Alternatively, you might place each hand on a pile of books positioned beside your ankles until you feel you are ready to stretch right back and hold your feet. As the joints in your spine regain flexibility you will be able to bend so far back that you can see the wall behind your head.

In the backbends the whole front of the body stretches over the framework provided by the spine and the rib cage. Keeping the thighs and the trunk stretching up throughout the pose, the breastbone lifting high, and the shoulders pressing back enables you to bend the spine still further.

Points to Watch

- Keep your shins and ankles pressing down onto the mat and your body lifting up from the knees throughout the pose.

- As you bend your head back, close your mouth, and breathe normally as you hold the pose.

- Do not allow your hips to sink back onto your heels—keep your tailbone pressing in.

- Take care: if you feel any strain or pain during this Level 3 pose, unwind by reversing the step sequence, and rest.

Camel pose analyzed

The details shown here help you achieve a full stretch in step 2 of the camel pose on page 179.

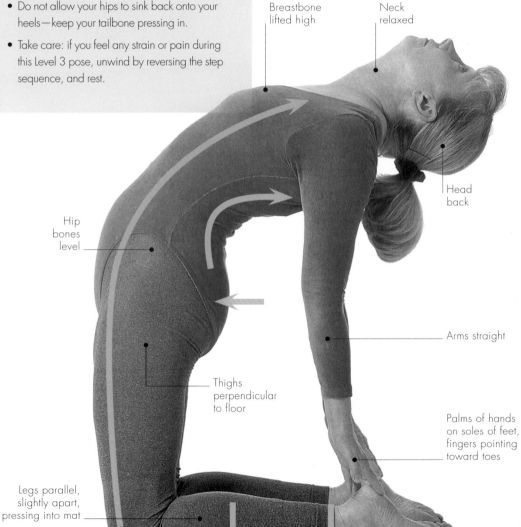

Breastbone lifted high

Neck relaxed

Head back

Hip bones level

Thighs perpendicular to floor

Arms straight

Palms of hands on soles of feet, fingers pointing toward toes

Legs parallel, slightly apart, pressing into mat

BOW

The bow pose or **dhanurasana** is a floor pose in which you stretch your whole body back and hold your ankles with your hands, so your body forms a bow shape with your arms as the bowstring. This is an extreme stretch, a demanding pose which, in time, will restore elasticity to the spine.

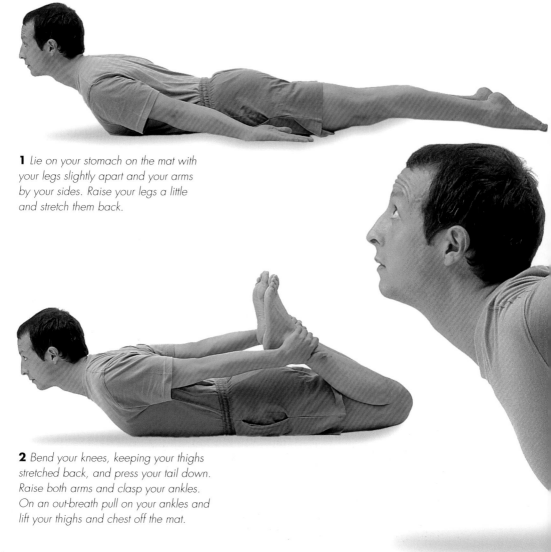

1 *Lie on your stomach on the mat with your legs slightly apart and your arms by your sides. Raise your legs a little and stretch them back.*

2 *Bend your knees, keeping your thighs stretched back, and press your tail down. Raise both arms and clasp your ankles. On an out-breath pull on your ankles and lift your thighs and chest off the mat.*

3 *Raise your head a little more, directing your gaze forward, and lift your shins higher breathing normally and without straining, for up to 10 seconds.*

Finish & rest
Breathe out, release your ankles, lower your legs and trunk to the mat, and rest.

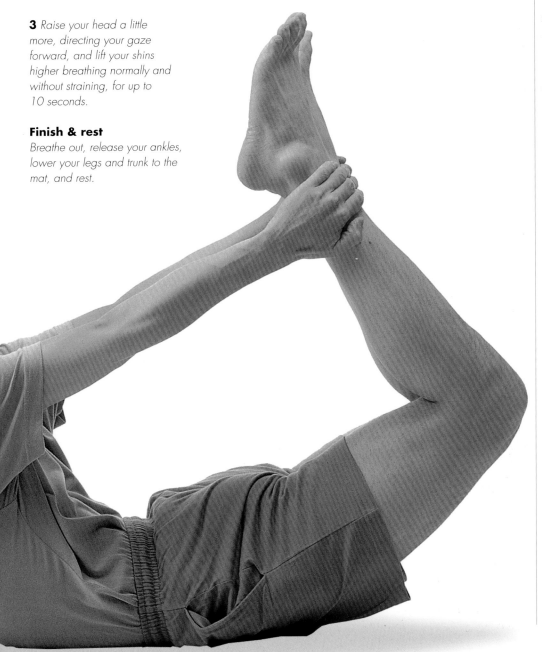

An Extreme Stretch

The bow pose on pages 182–83 gives the trunk and spine an extreme stretch, extending the front of the body as well as bending the back to its fullest extent. As in the camel pose on pages 178–81, pressing the tail in and the pelvis into the floor gives you the impetus you need to raise your legs off the mat, and stretching them up helps you hold them in position. And when you are holding the pose, pressing down in this way—a technique known as challenge and resistance—will enable you to bend your back a little more, and stretch from hips to breastbone. Pull on your ankles to lift your trunk and thighs higher.

Achieving lift

If you find it difficult at first to catch your ankles, practice the pose without lifting your legs off the mat. Begin by just stretching your arms back toward your ankles, then gradually raise your head and then your chest off the mat, and then work on raising your legs at the same time. Working in this way will improve the stretch on your trunk and legs, and make your spine more flexible. Then, when you can achieve more movement you can work on holding your ankles and lifting higher.

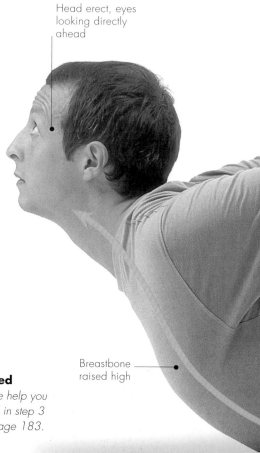

Head erect, eyes looking directly ahead

Breastbone raised high

Bow pose analyzed
The details shown here help you achieve the backbend in step 3 of the bow pose on page 183.

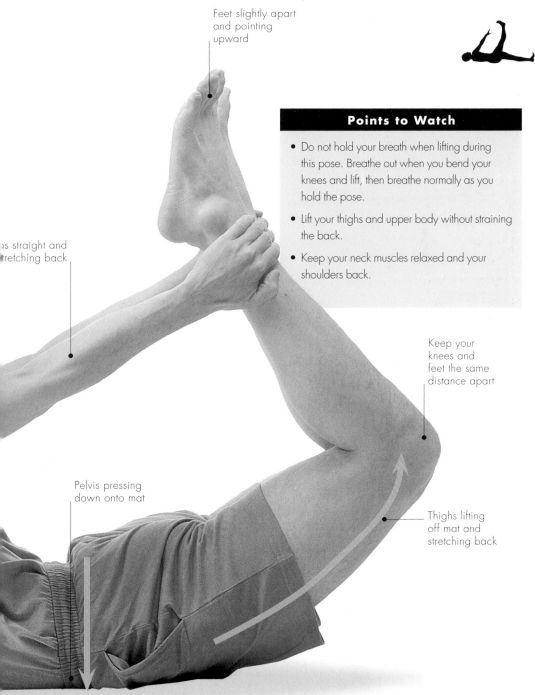

Feet slightly apart and pointing upward

...s straight and ...retching back

Pelvis pressing down onto mat

Keep your knees and feet the same distance apart

Thighs lifting off mat and stretching back

Points to Watch

- Do not hold your breath when lifting during this pose. Breathe out when you bend your knees and lift, then breathe normally as you hold the pose.

- Lift your thighs and upper body without straining the back.

- Keep your neck muscles relaxed and your shoulders back.

SHOULDER STAND & PLOW

The shoulder stand, **salamba sarvangasana**, and the plow or **halasana** may be performed separately, but here they are shown together as a sequence of movements. Before you begin, position a chair so that when you lie on the mat its seat is a little more than arm's length away, behind your head.

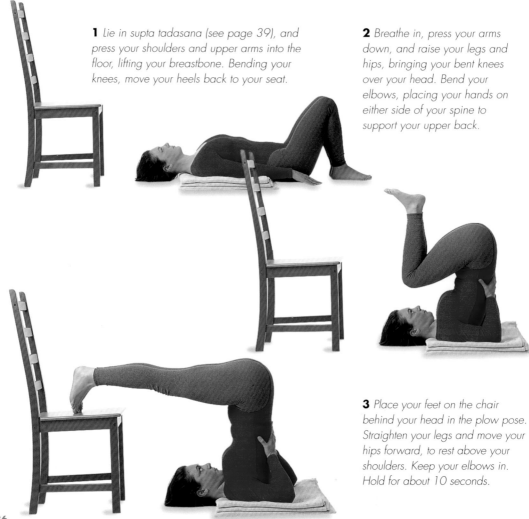

1 *Lie in supta tadasana (see page 39), and press your shoulders and upper arms into the floor, lifting your breastbone. Bending your knees, move your heels back to your seat.*

2 *Breathe in, press your arms down, and raise your legs and hips, bringing your bent knees over your head. Bend your elbows, placing your hands on either side of your spine to support your upper back.*

3 *Place your feet on the chair behind your head in the plow pose. Straighten your legs and move your hips forward, to rest above your shoulders. Keep your elbows in. Hold for about 10 seconds.*

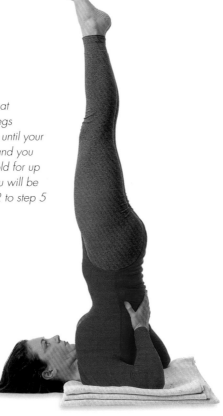

4 *Bend your knees, point them at the ceiling, and keeping your legs together, slowly straighten them until your feet are above your shoulders and you are doing a shoulder stand. Hold for up to 5 minutes. (With practice you will be able to do the pose from step 2 to step 5 without the use of a chair.)*

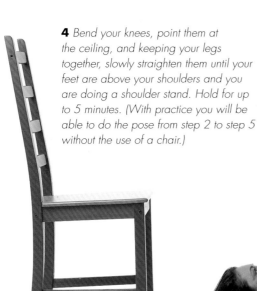

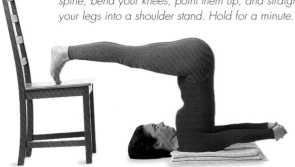

5 *Bend your knees, lower them toward your head, place your feet on the chair, then straighten your legs. Releasing your hands, interlock your fingers and stretch your arms along the floor behind your back. Now bend your elbows and place your hands either side of your spine, bend your knees, point them up, and straighten your legs into a shoulder stand. Hold for a minute.*

Finish & rest

Keeping your legs together, exhale, bend your knees and lower them toward your head, stretch your arms along the floor behind your back, pressing them down for control as you lower your hips to the floor. Rest with your legs bent.

Introducing Inverted Poses

Inverted poses have always been considered important in yoga because of their health-giving qualities. By stimulating blood and lymph circulation, they increase vitality.

Balance & control

Accurate alignment is important in these poses. Your head must be at right angles to your shoulders and not turned to either side. Stretching your arms toward your feet and pressing your shoulders and arms down lifts your breastbone and helps you maintain balance and control. When in the plow pose, interlocking your fingers and stretching your arms along the floor keeps your upper arms close and parallel to each other, giving you more control.

Keep your legs together throughout, and when you raise your body into a shoulder stand, stretch your thighs up so your ankles, hips, and shoulders are all in one plane. As you lower your legs into the plow pose, move your hips away from your head. When your feet touch the chair seat, straighten your bent knees, then move your hips forward toward your head so they lie above your shoulders,

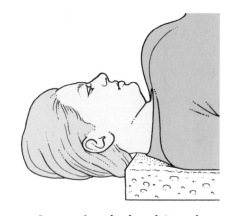

Supporting the head & neck
Begin both poses lying on your back, your upper body raised on three or four folded blankets or four foam blocks. This provides essential support for your neck.

tuck your toes under the insteps, and stretch your thighs up to straighten your legs even more.

Lowering the feet to a chair seat, placed at least an arm's length behind your head, is a good way of learning the plow pose. When you feel confident, attempt the full pose, lowering your feet to the mat.

Warning

Never practice this pose without raising your shoulders on foam blocks or three or four folded blankets, with your head lower. Do not do shoulder stands if you have high blood pressure or weakness or injury of the upper back, neck, or head. Women should avoid inverted poses when menstruating. Tie long hair back before practicing inverted poses.

Points to Watch

- In both poses, position your raised hips and trunk above your shoulders.
- Keep your sitting bones stretching away from your shoulders, your tail pressing in, and your thighs tucked back.
- Do not turn your head while in an inverted pose.
- Breathe normally throughout, lifting and lowering your body on an out-breath.

Shoulder stand analyzed

Check each of the points below for the shoulder stand on page 187.

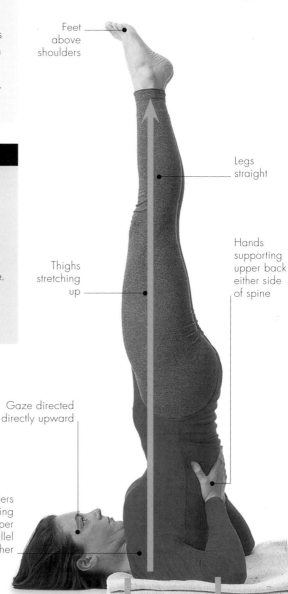

Feet above shoulders

Legs straight

Hands supporting upper back either side of spine

Thighs stretching up

Gaze directed directly upward

Shoulders pressing down, upper arms parallel to each other

189

SHOULDER STAND VARIATIONS
When you have learned the shoulder stand and the plow, and you feel confident with them, vary your practice with these poses on the same theme. These pages show three poses from a sequence of more than 20 which make up the **sarvangasana** cycle—asanas based on the shoulder stand on page 186–87. These three poses follow each other with no more than a brief rest.

Eka pada sarvangasana
Keeping your left leg stretching up strongly lower your right leg to the floor or a chair seat, keeping it straight. Hold for about 10–15 seconds, then raise it beside your left leg, stretching both legs up in a shoulder stand again. Then repeat, keeping your right leg stretching up and lowering your left leg to the chair seat, then stretch up in the shoulder stand.

Parsvaika pada sarvangasana
Stretch up in a shoulder stand and turn your right leg out at the hip joint. Keeping it straight, lower it diagonally to the floor, resting your right toes in line with your right shoulder. Hold for 10–15 seconds, then raise the leg into a shoulder stand. Repeat, lowering your left leg to the floor, and stretch up into a shoulder stand.

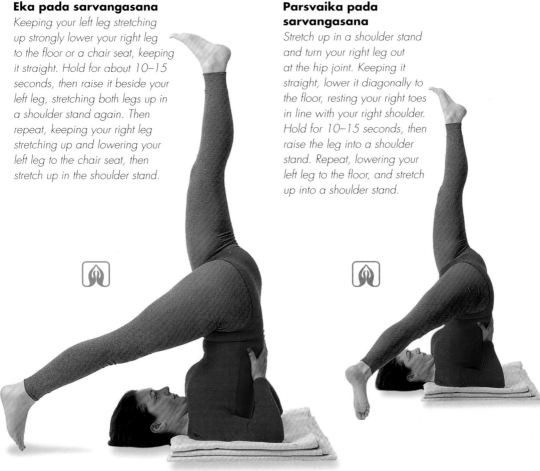

Supta konasana

1 Lift up in a strong shoulder stand, supporting your back with your hands. Exhale, bend your knees into plow pose (see page 186) but with your feet on the floor. Straighten your legs and spread them apart in a wide-legged plow pose.

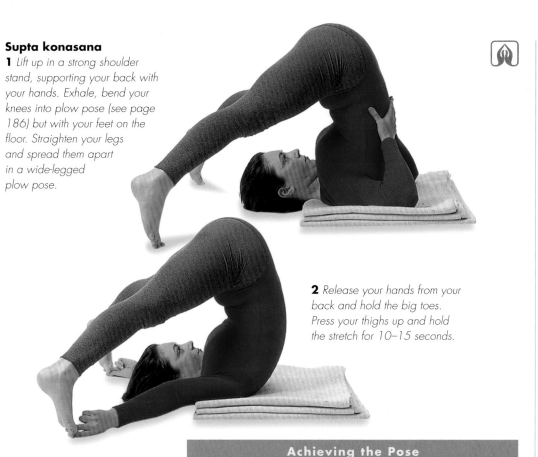

2 Release your hands from your back and hold the big toes. Press your thighs up and hold the stretch for 10–15 seconds.

Finish & rest

Release your toes, support your back with your hands, walk your feet together into plow pose. Then on an out-breath, bend your knees and return to a shoulder stand. Keeping your legs together, bend your knees, stretch your arms along the floor, and pressing your arms down, lower your hips and trunk to the floor. Rest with your knees bent.

Achieving the Pose

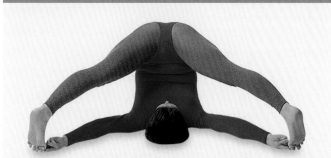

Breathe out before spreading your feet as wide apart as you can at the end of step 1. Grasp your big toes between the thumb and first fingers of each hand. If you cannot reach your toes, hold your ankles or your calves.

Working on Shoulder Stands

These three poses are all fairly advanced and you should try them only when you feel confident with the shoulder stand and plow pose on pages 186–87. Bear in mind that these are all balancing exercises, and since they are inverted poses it is important to be confident about lowering your body to the floor. The best way to learn the one-leg shoulder stand, eka pada sarvangasana, is to lower one leg onto a chair as you did in the plow. As you gain confidence, you can take your leg still further down— to two foam blocks, perhaps, and then to the floor. Support your upper back with your hands throughout the pose.

Focus on alignment

In eka pada sarvangasana the upward-stretching leg must face forward, toward your head, but in parsvaika pada sarvangasana, the diagonal leg-stretch to the floor, you turn your right leg out from the hip before lowering it. In both poses, keep both legs stiff as you lower one to the chair seat or the floor, and keep your hips level: as the right leg comes down, lift the right hip, and vice versa. Remember to lower and raise your legs on an out-breath.

Supta konasana on page 191 combines a wide-legged stretch with the plow. Like all inverted poses, its aims are to raise the trunk and hips above the shoulders and to stretch the whole body. Supta konasana is an extreme stretch, but like all the exercises in this section, once you have practiced it and can do it easily, it becomes a calming, relaxing pose.

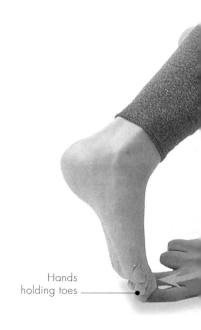

Hands
holding toes

Supta konasana analyzed

The image below analyzes supta konasana—
the wide-legged plow pose—on page 191,
but most of the details relate to all three
shoulder stand variations on pages 190–91.

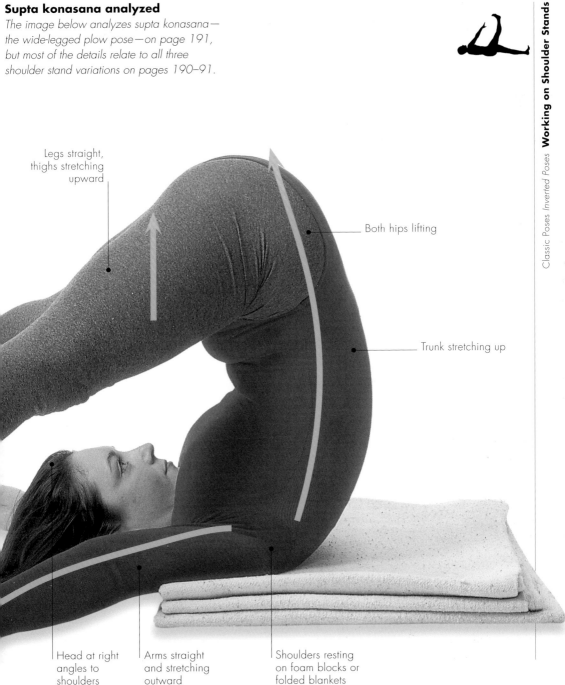

Legs straight,
thighs stretching
upward

Both hips lifting

Trunk stretching up

Head at right
angles to
shoulders

Arms straight
and stretching
outward

Shoulders resting
on foam blocks or
folded blankets

SHOULDER EXERCISES
Although some people exercise their shoulders regularly because their work demands it, most people's lives are largely sedentary nowadays, and this encourages rounded shoulders. This chapter ends with two exercises—hand clasp or **gomukhasana**, and arm twist or **garudasana**—to stretch the shoulders, arms, and hands, and open the chest.

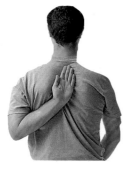

Hand clasp
1 *Inhale, bend your left arm up behind your back, moving your forearm as close as you can to your spine, and the backs of your fingers touching your spine as high up as you can reach.*

3 *Stretch your left elbow down to bring your left hand further up; and stretch your right elbow toward the ceiling to bring your right hand further down, then clasp your hands. Hold for 20 seconds.*

Repeat & finish
Release your hands, raise your right arm above your head, and lower both arms to your sides, then repeat steps 2 and 3, bending your right arm up behind your back and raising your left arm.

2 *Keeping the back of your left hand against your spine, lift your right arm above your head, turn it at the shoulder until the palm faces behind you, and bend it back toward the fingers of your left hand.*

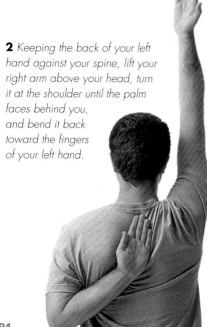

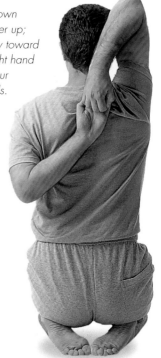

Arm twist

1 *Breathe in, stretch both arms out to the sides, and as you breathe out, swing your arms rapidly forward as if you are hugging yourself, crossing the right upper arm over the left at chest level.*

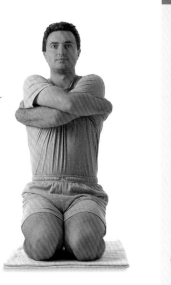

Twisting the Hands

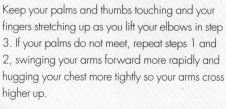

Keep your palms and thumbs touching and your fingers stretching up as you lift your elbows in step 3. If your palms do not meet, repeat steps 1 and 2, swinging your arms forward more rapidly and hugging your chest more tightly so your arms cross higher up.

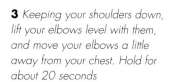

3 *Keeping your shoulders down, lift your elbows level with them, and move your elbows a little away from your chest. Hold for about 20 seconds*

Repeat & finish

Release your hands and repeat steps 1–3, this time crossing the left upper arm over the right at chest level.

2 *Bending both arms, bring the backs of your hands together, fingers pointing up, then move your left hand toward you and your right hand slightly back, and move your hands together until the palms touch.*

Mobilizing the Shoulders

Sitting at a desk, reading on a train, or reclining to watch television fill hours of many people's lives, and they do not realize how hunched their shoulders have become. In free moments, try these simple exercises to stretch your shoulders, arms, and hands. Like namaste on page 94, which is an integral part of the side-stretch, parsvottanasana, the shoulder exercises on pages 194–95 can be an integral part of a pose, or alternatively practiced alone. Begin by standing in a good tadasana (see pages 42–43), or sitting cross-legged in sukhasana (see page 38), or kneeling in the hero pose or virasana (see page 107). Before beginning, concentrate for a moment on lifting the spine and stretching across the upper chest, broadening your shoulders, and flattening your shoulder blades against your ribs.

Hand clasp

The hand clasp, gomukhasana, pulls the shoulders firmly back and stretches the upper arms. The key to this pose is to move the upward-stretching hand and arm as close to the center of the back as is possible. The aim of this pose is to

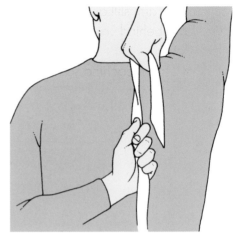

Joining the hands
If your shoulders are stiff, you may be unable to move your arm far toward the spine in the hand clasp, so that only your fingers meet. The answer is to hold a belt and walk both hands along it, toward each other.

clasp the hands together, and for that the upward-stretching hand needs to reach high up the back, between the shoulder blades. The downward-stretching arm also needs to be aligned accurately. As you stretch it up in step 2, keep it well back, touching the side of your head; and when you have turned it so that the hand faces behind you,

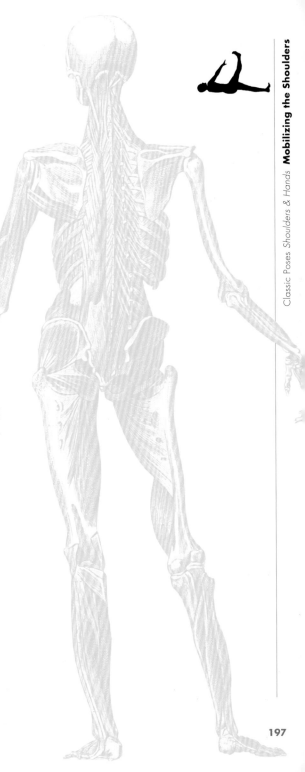

keep the upper arm still as you bend the forearm down behind your back. Letting the elbow form a wing out to the side will prevent it from reaching so far.

Arm twist

Some yoga courses tell you to begin the hand twist, garudasana, by simply crossing your upper arms, but this graceful pose will be easier if you begin by throwing your arms around your chest as if giving yourself a bear-hug. That makes it easier to cross the upper arms high up.

When you bring your palms together after crossing your arms in step 2, you will be able to see your thumbs in front of your nose, the fingers stretching away behind them. Keep them at that height, but move them a little way from your body, keeping your shoulders down, and you will increase the stretch on your upper arms.

HAND EXERCISES

Most of what we do with our hands involves moving and closing them. This exercise stretches them, exercises the joints, and makes them more flexible. It improves circulation in the fingers on cold days, and is said to be a good preventive and a therapy for repetitive strain injury (RSI) and mild arthritis.

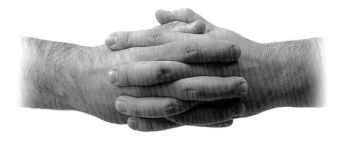

Interlocking fingers

1 *Clasp your hands in front of you by interlocking your fingers so that your right thumb lies on top.*

2 *Turn your clasped hands palms outward, and stretch your arms forward.*

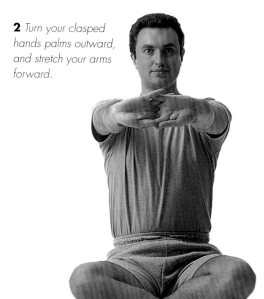

3 *Keeping your fingers interlocked, stretch your arms up above your head, then back so that your upper arms lie either side of your head, brushing your ears.*

Repeat & rest

Repeat steps 1 and 2, this time interlocking your fingers so your left thumb lies uppermost.

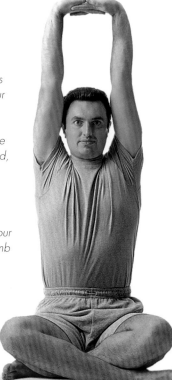

Finger twister

1 Hold your two hands up parallel to your chest, palms facing down, tips of your middle fingers just touching, then turn the palm of the left hand up. Stretch the index finger and the little finger of each hand out to the sides, then bend the two middle fingers of the left hand up and the two middle fingers of the right hand down. Now move your hands closer together, sliding the little finger of your right hand across the index finger of your left hand, and your right index finger across your left little finger.

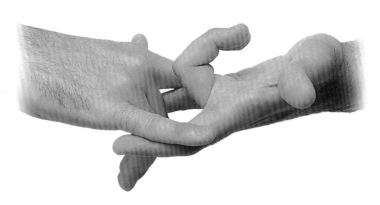

2 Turn your left hand toward you, and straighten the two middle fingers of your left hand so they lie across the knuckle of your right index finger. Raise your right thumb and press it down on the tips of the two middle fingers. Pause to open your palms.

3 Now straighten the two middle fingers of your right hand, and stretching them away from you, tuck your left thumb beneath the tips. To achieve this you may need to move your hands a little further apart, widening the gap in the center. Hold your hands up and if you have achieved the finger twist you should be able to see through the gap between the index and middle fingers.

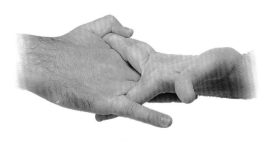

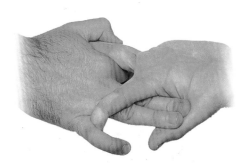

Flexing the Hands

We use our marvelously flexible hands all the time, but we rarely exercise them. We contract and relax sets of muscles to put things down and pick them up, but few of the everyday movements we make involve stretching the fingers and bending them outward, bending the wrist back, or stretching the palms. Like every part of the skeleton, the hands have joints and muscles that need to be exercised to keep them supple. If you injure your hand you need to restore flexibility to the muscles, and hand and wrist exercises may reduce the effects of diseases affecting the joints, such as arthritis, and perhaps prevent them.

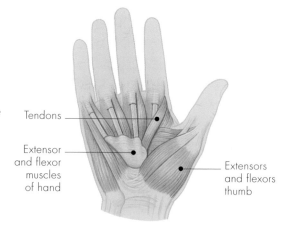

Tendons

Extensor and flexor muscles of hand

Extensors and flexors thumb

Hand muscles

More than 40 muscles, some of them tiny, move the fingers, thumb, and wrist to make the hand an extraordinarily flexible instrument.

Hand flexors

Several yoga poses incorporate hand exercises. For example, in the side-stretch (parsvottanasana on pages 94–97) the hands form the prayer pose or namaste behind your back. This movement stretches the palms and fingers laterally and longitudinally, and flexes the wrist as you turn your hands inward. The shoulder exercises on pages 194–97 also stretch the hands. You can practice hand exercises to fill free moments.

Finger twister

If you find you can do it easily, move your fingers closer together at the start to give them less space to maneuver. It is a great cold weather exercise since it improves the circulation to the fingers.

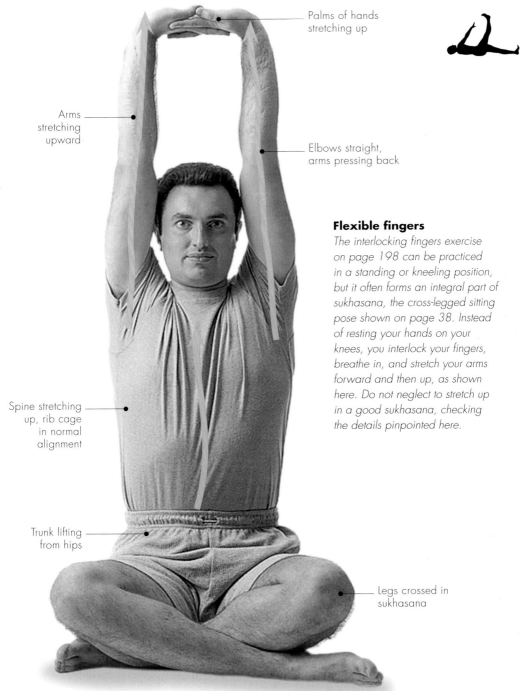

Palms of hands
stretching up

Arms
stretching
upward

Elbows straight,
arms pressing back

Flexible fingers

*The interlocking fingers exercise
on page 198 can be practiced
in a standing or kneeling position,
but it often forms an integral part of
sukhasana, the cross-legged sitting
pose shown on page 38. Instead
of resting your hands on your
knees, you interlock your fingers,
breathe in, and stretch your arms
forward and then up, as shown
here. Do not neglect to stretch up
in a good sukhasana, checking
the details pinpointed here.*

Spine stretching
up, rib cage
in normal
alignment

Trunk lifting
from hips

Legs crossed in
sukhasana

PLANNING
YOUR PRACTICE

This final chapter helps you plan your own future yoga practices based on the 50 classic poses illustrated and described step-by-step in this book. The following two pages give guidelines for designing a program to suit your particular needs. The pages that follow show three short sample programs. Try the first program when you are ready to progress from exercises for beginners to those presenting a slightly higher level of difficulty (see page 206 for full icon key); and the second when you eventually feel ready to try more advanced poses. The chapter ends with a short practice for whenever you feel tired or stressed.

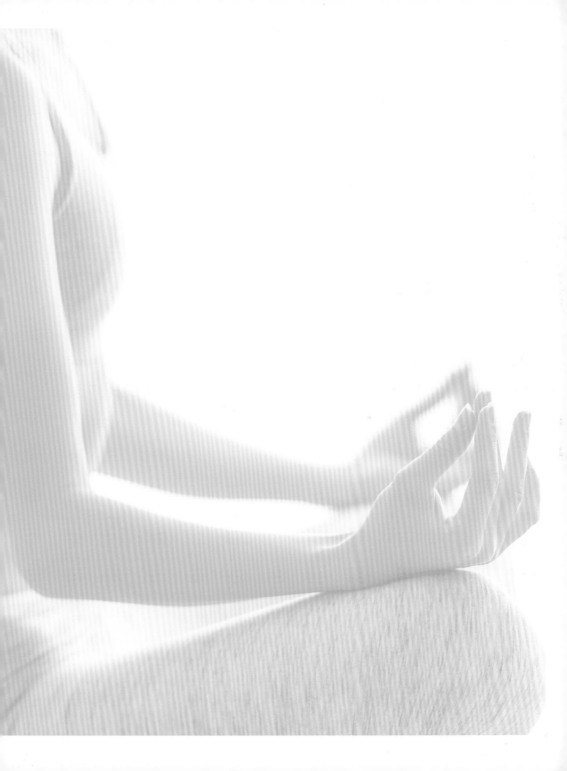

Designing Your Yoga Course

The important principle in yoga is always to progress at your own pace. Start with the beginner's poses in Chapter 3, and as long as you practice regularly, concentrating on the details of each exercise, do not worry if you prefer to stay with the ten poses shown on those pages for some weeks, until you can do them well.

Expanding your repertoire

You will soon want to introduce new poses into your practice, and this book is planned to enable you to progress in whichever way suits you best. The poses in Chapter 4 are grouped into different types of exercise—standing poses, sitting poses, floor poses, and so on. Each is graded according to its level of difficulty. Beginners usually start with the standing poses, but you could try a sitting pose, a floor pose, such as the downward-facing dog pose on pages 130–31, or even the cross-legged sitting twist on pages 158–59.

There are few rules in yoga, simply because everyone's body is different and everyone has different levels of capability, so if your body is quite flexible and you want to try one of the higher-level poses, do not feel you must wait. However, it is a good idea to begin with a simple pose.

Resting time

Between poses, the muscles and joints need a chance to recover from stretching, the breathing must be allowed to return to normal, and the mind needs to recenter itself. For example, after a standing pose, return to tadasana (pages 42–43), and to dandasana (page 106) after a sitting pose. Rest on your back at the end of a floor pose with your knees raised to your chest and your hands clasped around them. Sit on your heels after a backbend, and relax with your legs bent after a shoulder stand.

Do make your favorite poses a part of your practice—after all, you should enjoy yoga—but include a good mix of poses in your program. Start with standing poses since they tone your muscles and boost your circulation, waking you up, followed by calming sitting or floor poses, which give muscles and joints a good stretch. Then exercise the spine with an energizing sitting twist followed by a backbend. Leave new and less familiar poses until last—finish with the shoulder stand and plow (pages 186–87), for instance. And end with the corpse pose, savasana (pages 64–65), to rest your body and mind completely.

Standing Poses

These are the five basic standing poses in the order in which they should be practiced: hold the standing poses for 10–15 seconds each side at first, then repeat as often as you like. Breathe normally through the nose.

1 Triangle   pages 46–47

2 Extended side angle   pages 50–51

3 Warrior II   pages 78–79

4 Warrior I   pages 82–83

5 Side-stretch   pages 94–95

A SECOND-LEVEL PROGRAM

These four pages present a program of second-level poses. You can tackle them at any stage, but to master them you will need a degree of flexibility, especially in the hips, for they are mainly sitting poses. If you have been practicing yoga for three to four months you should have that flexibility; if not, you may need the help of foam blocks or folded blankets. This program should last about an hour, but work at your own speed. Aim to practice it at least once a week.

Levels of Difficulty

Within each category the poses appear in order of increasing complexity, and each has an icon

 BEGINNERS for complete beginners

INTERMEDIATE slightly more advanced—you have worked through Chapter 3 at least once

ADVANCED more advanced poses to use when your body has gained some flexibility

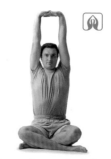

1 Cross-legged sitting
sukhasana with parvatasana,
pages 38 and 201

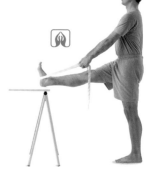

2 Extended leg-stretch I
utthita hasta padangusthasana,
page 70

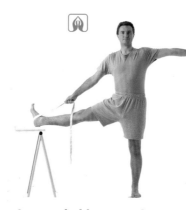

3 Extended leg-stretch II
utthita hasta padangusthasana II,
page 71

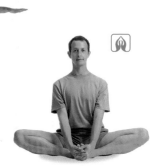

4 Cobbler
baddha konasana,
page 110

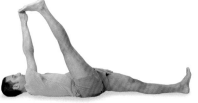

5 Floor leg-stretch I
supta padangusthasana I,
page 146–47

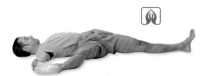

6 Floor leg-stretch II
supta padangusthasana II,
page 147

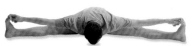

7 Angled leg-stretch
upavistha konasana,
page 111

8 Head-to-knee pose
janu sirsasana,
pages 114–15

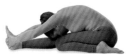

9 Three-limbed pose
*triang mukhaikapada
paschimottanasana,*
pages 118–19

10 Sitting forward bend
paschimottanasana,
pages 122–23

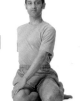

11 Mermaid I
Bharadvajasana I,
pages 162–63

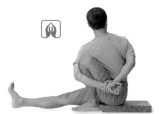

12 Sage
Marichyasana I,
page 166

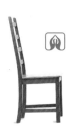

13 Shoulder stand & plow
salamba sarvangasana and halasana,
pages 186–87

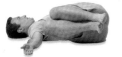

14 Revolving abdomen
jathara parivartanasana,
pages 138–39

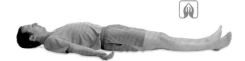

15 Corpse
savasana I,
pages 64–65

Concentrating on Sitting Poses

Every practice needs to begin with a passive pose to quiet and focus the mind. This program starts with cross-legged sitting, a restful sitting pose in which you concentrate on stretching your arms up in parvatasana. An invigorating standing pose follows to stretch and tone your legs. As you work through the program you may find you need to rest briefly between the stretches by lying for a few seconds with your knees clasped to your chest. Between leg-stretches you concentrate on opening the hips. The second part of the practice works on the back in a succession of forward bends and twists.

Go as far as you can with each pose, supporting yourself whenever you need to on a ledge, a chair back or seat, foam blocks, or piles of books. For the safety of your neck, never attempt the shoulder stand (pose 13) without resting your shoulders and upper arms on folded blankets or foam blocks so your head lies back below their level.

1 Cross-legged sitting

Begin the the second-level program quietly in sukhasana (page 38) with your arms stretched above your head in parvatasana (page 201). Hold the pose for about 20 seconds, stretching up throughout.

2 & 3 Extended leg-stretches

Stretch your hip joints and wake up the muscles of your hips and legs with utthita hasta padangusthasana I and II (pages 70–71). Aim to hold the pose for up to a minute.

4 Cobbler

Now sit with your back against a wall and relax into baddha konasana (page 110), clasping your feet with your hands. You may want to hold this pose for more than a minute.

5 & 6 Floor leg-stretches

Return to leg-stretches—supta padangusthasana I and II (pages 146–47) performed lying on the mat. Raise each leg in turn, holding the stretch for up to a minute. End with a few seconds in a resting position.

7 Angled leg-stretch

The angled leg-stretch upavistha konasana (page 111) stretches both legs out to the sides. Remember to breathe out as you lean forward. Hold for 20 seconds, and finish in a resting pose.

8 Head-to-knee pose

Janu sirsasana (pages 114–15) marks a change of position following the two leg-stretches. Perform the pose on the right side, then on the left. Hold for about 30 seconds each side. This is a resting pose, so relax into it.

9 Three-limbed pose

Keep your hips level as you extend your trunk forward in triang mukhaikapada paschimottanasana (pages 118–19). This second sitting forward bend is a relaxing pose, so hold it for 30 seconds on each side.

10 Sitting forward bend

End this sequence of three forward bends with paschimottanasana (pages 122–23), stretching your trunk forward with both legs extended. This is a restful pose. Hold it for up to 1 minute, if you can.

11 Mermaid I

Follow a succession of forward bends with Bharadvajasana I (pages 162–63), rotating your spine first to the right, then to the left. Hold each twist for up to 30 seconds.

12 Sage

Marichyasana (page 166) gives the back a satisfying stretch. Hold it for at least 20 seconds on each side, then rest in a kneeling position for a few seconds.

13 Shoulder stand & plow

Two inverted poses, salamba sarvangasana and halasana (pages 186–87), carried out in tandem for about 3 minutes, will be invigorating.

14 Revolving abdomen

In this last active pose—jathara parivartanasana (pages 138–39)—the legs swing to one side, then the other, exercising the spine. Practice for up to 20 seconds on each side.

15 Corpse

Finish with a 10-minute rest in the corpse pose (savasana I, pages 64–65).

A THIRD-LEVEL PROGRAM This program includes some of the basic poses from Chapter 3, such as the triangle and the kneeling forward bend. One of the reasons for this is that the body, especially the legs, needs to be strong for the more complex poses, and the standing poses at the beginning of the program are chosen to give essential preparatory stretches. The program concentrates on energizing: the standing poses at the beginning wake the body up, and the backbends stimulate the mind and body. It focuses on backbends, which mobilize the spine, giving it an extreme stretch. The sequence should take about 75 minutes, although it is important not to hurry. Repeat the program at least once a week.

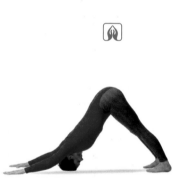

1 Downward-facing dog
adho mukha svanasana,
pages 130–31

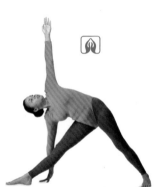

2 Triangle
utthita trikonasana,
pages 46–47

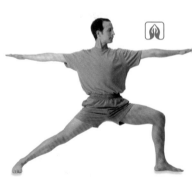

3 Warrior II
virabhadrasana II,
pages 78–79

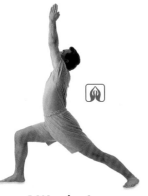

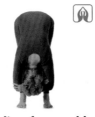

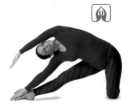

4 Warrior I
virabhadrasana I,
pages 82–83

5 Standing forward bend
uttanasana I,
page 75

6 Gate
parighasana,
pages 134–35

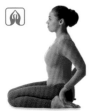

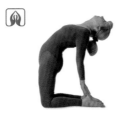

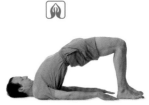

7 Hero
virasana,
page 107

8 Camel
ustrasana,
pages 178–79

9 Bridge
sarvangasana setu bandha,
pages 170–71

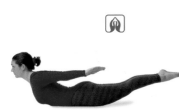

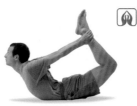

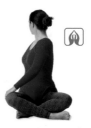

10 Locust
salabhasana,
pages 174–74

11 Bow
dhanurasana,
pages 182–83

12 Cross-legged twist
sukhasana twist,
pages 158–59

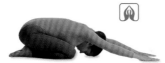

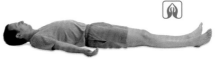

13 Kneeling
forward bend,
page 54

14 Corpse
savasana I,
pages 64–65

Concentrating on Backbends

Although this is a stimulating practice, it is a good idea to begin with a few minutes sitting cross-legged or in the hero pose to quiet the mind. It incorporates some demanding poses, but the program is punctuated by restful postures, such as calming forward bends.

In the second half of the practice you work on the spine in a sequence of backbends, which elongate the whole trunk from the groin to the neck and extend the spine. The stretching opens up the chest and the front of the body. The backbends and twists give an extreme stretch, so you may need to rest briefly, sitting back on your heels, perhaps, or lying on the floor with your knees drawn up to your chest and your hands clasped over your shins after a particularly intense effort. As always, end the program with a 5–10 minute rest in the corpse pose. Afterward you will still find that the program has had an invigorating effect.

1 Downward-facing dog

Begin with the muscle-toning, body-stretching adho mukha svanasana (pages 130–31), which relaxes the heart. Hold for up to one minute.

2 Triangle

Utthita trikonasana (pages 46–47) is included here to strengthen the legs. Hold the pose for up to 20 seconds on the right and the left.

3 Warrior II

A sequence of wake-up standing poses continues with virabhadrasana II (pages 78–79). Hold the pose for up to 20 seconds each side.

4 Warrior I

Concentrate on stretching up in virabhadrasana I (pages 82–83). Hold for a maximum of 15 seconds each side.

5 Standing forward bend

The standing poses end with uttanasana I (page 75), which slows the heartbeat and calms the nerves. Keeping your legs, bend from the hips. Hold for a minute, breathing normally through the nose.

6 Gate
Parighasana (pages 134–35) introduces a short sequence of kneeling and sitting postures at the heart of this practice. This pose stretches each side of the body in turn. Hold for up to 10 seconds on each side, feeling the stretch.

7 Hero
When performed correctly, so that your sitting bones touch the floor between your feet, virasana (page 107) stretches the feet, the ankles, and the knees. This is a relaxing pose, so hold it for more than a minute.

8 Camel
The first in the sequence of backbends, ustrasana (pages 178–79) stretches the whole spine up as well as back. Hold for up to 10 seconds, then rest, sitting back on your heels.

9 Bridge
For this second backbend, arch your back in sarvangasana setu bandha (pages 170–71). Hold the pose for up to 10 seconds, then rest with your legs bent and your feet on the mat.

10 Locust
In salabhasana (pages 174–75) you lift your legs and upper body, giving your spine an extreme stretch. Hold for up to 10 seconds.

11 Bow
Dhanurasana (pages 182–83), the last in the backbend sequence, exercises the joints of the spine. Hold for up to 10 seconds.

12 Cross-legged twist
The sukhasana twist (pages 158–59) rotates the spine, moving it in a different direction from the backbends. Hold for up to 15 seconds.

13 Kneeling forward bend
This bend (page 54) rests the back after the twist that precedes it. Hold the pose for two minutes or more.

14 Corpse
Five to ten minutes of full relaxation in savasana I (pages 64–65) is essential after the effort demanded by this practice.

EASING STRESS & FATIGUE
This short practice makes an excellent pick-me-up after a hard day's work, whenever you are tired or feel stressed or anxious, or when you just need to give yourself a little tender loving care. It is a simple program of four relaxing postures, intended to be used as remedy for fatigue of any kind, because it will enable you to refresh your mind and body with minimum effort. The program works because the poses are passive—that is, although you make the effort to stretch in one pose, lift in another, or just concentrate your mind in a third, you are not actively moving or even stretching intensively. This program is estimated to take around 20–25 minutes, but relax in each pose for as long as you feel you need to.

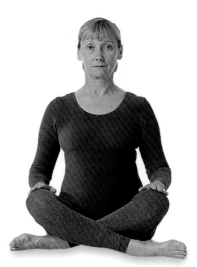

1 Cross-legged sitting
Calm your mind by sitting cross-legged in sukhasana (page 38) for a minute or two, your eyes closed. Support your back by sitting on a foam block against a wall. Breathe normally through the nose and listen to your breathing pattern.

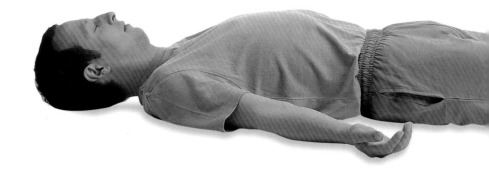

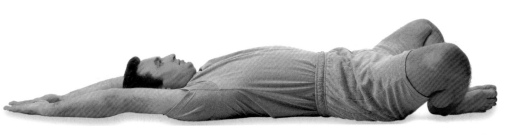

2 Cobbler floor pose
Rest your back in supta baddha konasana (pages 126–27). By now, your mind should be calm and your body relaxing. This posture is especially helpful to women during menstruation.

3 Extended leg-stretch
Relieve aching legs by lying on your back and extending them in urdhva prasarita padasana (pages 62–63) while supporting them against a wall. This pose may also alleviate an aching back.

4 Corpse pose
All practices end in the corpse pose (pages 64–65). You should now be completely relaxed. Concentrate on breathing in normally, but taking long, slow out-breaths.

GLOSSARY

Asana (pronounced "ah-sna") A yoga pose or posture.

Extend To extend a part of the body is to straighten or to stretch it.

Flex To flex a part of the body is to contract muscles in order to bend it.

Groin The groove between the bottom of the abdomen and the top of the thigh. The two groins slope out from the center of the pubic area and upward.

Hatha yoga A pathway to achieving universal wholeness or samadhi through practicing asanas, breathing, and cleansing processes; a classic school of yoga which evolved about 1,000 years ago.

Iyengar yoga A school or style of yoga founded by the Indian teacher, B.K.S. Iyengar.

Mantra Sacred words or sounds, such as "om," used to concentrate the mind.

Passive pose A yoga posture in which you stretch, but do not change position.

Pranayamas Energy-expanding techniques, including special breathing exercises.

Pratyahara Control of the senses.

Trunk The central part of the body, excluding the head, the arms, and the legs. Also called the torso.

Yoga Oneness or union.

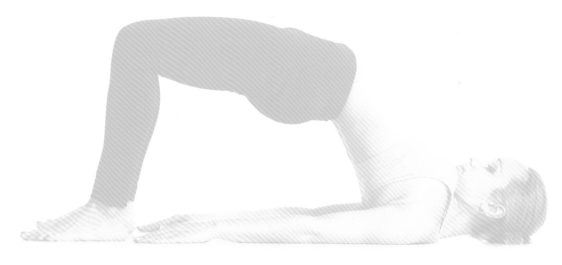

The Asanas

SANSKRIT NAME	ENGLISH NAME	SANSKRIT NAME	ENGLISH NAME
adho mukha svanasana	downward-facing dog pose	sarvangasana	shoulder stand
anantasana	side-reclining leg lift pose	sarvangasana setu bandha	bridge
		savasana	corpse poses
ardha chandrasana	half-moon pose	sukhasana	cross-legged sitting; cross-legged twist
ardha navasana	half-boat pose		
baddha konasana	cobbler pose	supta baddha konasana	cobbler floor pose
Bharadvajasana	mermaid pose		
chaturanga andasana	four-limbed rod pose	supta konasana pose	wide-legged plow
dandasana	rod pose	supta padangusthasana	floor leg-stretches
dhanurasana	bow	supta tadasana	lying-down mountain pose
eka pada sarvangasana	one-leg shoulder stand		
garudasana	arm twist	supta virasana	hero floor pose
gomukhasana	hand clasp	tadasana	standing mountain pose
halasana	plow		
janu sirsasana	head-to-knee pose	triang mukhaikapada paschimottanasana	three-limbed pose
jathara parivartanasana	revolving abdomen	upavistha konasana	angled leg-stretch
Marichyasana	sage pose	urdhva prasarita padasana	extended leg-stretch
parighasana	gate pose	ustrasana	camel pose
paripurna navasana	boat with oars	utkatasana	chair pose
parivrtta trikonasana	revolved triangle	uttanasana	standing forward bend
parsvaika pada sarvangasana	diagonal leg-stretch shoulder stand	utthita hasta padangusthasana	leg-stretches
parsvottanasana	side-stretch	utthita parsvakonasana	extended side-angle pose
parvatasana	interlocking fingers	utthita trikonasana	triangle pose
paschimottanasana	sitting forward bend	virabhadrasana	warrior pose
prasarita padottanasana	wide leg-stretch	virasana	hero pose
salabhasana	locust	vrksasana	tree pose
salamba sarvangasana	shoulder stand		

217

FURTHER READING

Yoga

Iyengar B.K.S. *B.K.S. Iyengar Yoga The Path to Holistic Health.* Dorling Kindersley, 2014.

Iyengar, B.K.S. *Iyengar Yoga For Beginners.* Dorling Kindersley, 2006.

Iyengar, B.K.S. *Light on Life: The Journey to Wholeness, Inner Peace and Ultimate Freedom.* Rodale, 2008.

Iyengar B.K.S. *Light on Yoga: The Definitive Guide to Yoga Practice.* Harper Thorsons, 2015.

Iyengar, Geeta S. *Yoga – A Gem for Women.* Timeless Books, 2002.

Iyengar, Geeta S. *Yoga in Action: Preliminary Course.* YOG, 2000.

Kent, Howard. *Yoga for the Disabled.* Sunrise Thorsons, 1985.

Mehta, Silva, Mira Mehta. *Yoga the Iyengar Way.* Dorling Kindersley, 1990.

Olkin, Silvia Klein. *Positive Pregnancy Fitness, A Guide to a More Comfortable Pregnancy and Easier Birth Through Exercise and Relaxation.* Avery Publications, 1996.

The Body

Hinkle, Carla Z. *Fundamentals of Anatomy and Movement.* Mosby, 1997.

Key, Sarah. *The Back Sufferer's Bible.* Telegraph Books, 2000.

Key, Sarah. *Body in Action.* BBC Books,1992.

Classic Yoga Texts

Bahm, Archie J. *The Yoga Sutras of Patañjali.* Asian Humanities Press, 1993.

Iyengar, B.K.S. *Core of the Yoga Sutras: The Definitive Guide to the Philosophy of Yoga.* Harper Thorsons, 2012.

Iyengar, B.K.S. *Light on Pranayama: The Definitive Guide to the Art of Breathing.* Harper Thorsons, 2013.

Iyengar, B.K.S. *Light on the Yoga Sutras of Patañjali.* Aquarian Press,1992.

Mascaro, Juan, (trans.). *The Bhagavad Gita.* Penguin Books, 1998.

Mascaro, Juan, (trans.). *The Upanishads.* Penguin Books, 1998.

Nikhilananda, S. (trans.). *The Upanishads.* Ramakrishna-Vivekananda Center, New York, 1993.

Yogananda, Pramahansa. *Autobiography of a Yogi.* Rider, 1991.

USEFUL ADDRESSES

JB Hypnotherapy
www.jb-hypnotherapy.co.uk
Information on experienced and qualified hypnotherapy and psychotherapy practitioner, Jennie Bittleston.

Australian Institute of Yoga Therapy
www.australianyogatherapy.com.au
The longest running yoga therapy organization in Australia who specialize in professional development programs for qualified yoga therapists.

B.K.S Iyengar Yoga
www.bksiyengar.com
The official website of B.K.S Iyengar Yoga detailing institutions and a directory of teachers around the world.

British Wheel of Yoga
www.bwy.org.uk
Information on yoga groups and organizations throughout the UK.

Centre for Mindfulness Research and Practice
Bangor University, Wales
www.bangor.ac.uk/mindfulness/
Information on one of the key mindfulness centres in Europe.

Divine Life Society
www.sivanandaonline.org
An organization aimed at promoting yoga worldwide.

Iyengar Yoga UK
www.iyengaryoga.org.uk

Iyengar Yoga Institute, London
www.iyi.org.uk
One of the first yoga studios in Europe, they provide practice, research, support, and training for Iyengar yoga students and teachers in London.

IYNAUS Iyengar National Association of the United States
www.iynaus.org
The website contains a list of regional associations throughout North America.

Sivananda Yoga
www.sivananda.org
The official website of the International Sivananda Yoga Vendanta Centers.

Yoga Journal
www.yogajournal.com
A magazine with useful information on all branches of yoga.

Yoga Site
www.yogasite.com
A general information website.

Yogaville
www.yogaville.org
The international headquarters of Integral Yoga.

United States Yoga Federation
www.usayoga.org
A nonprofit organization dedicated to promoting and developing yoga as a sport.

INDEX

ACKNOWLEDGMENTS

The publisher would like to thank Deborah Fielding
for reading and commenting on the text.

Special thanks go to Louise Beglin, Carla Carrington, Linda de Comarmond,
Fiona Grantham, Kay Macmullan, Ben Morgan, Maria Rivans, David Ronchetti,
and Arup Sen for help with photography.

With thanks to Dancia International, London for the kind loan of props.

PICTURE ACKNOWLEDGMENTS

Every effort has been made to trace copyright holders and obtain permission.
The publishers apologize for any omissions and would be pleased
to make any necessary changes at subsequent printings

Alamy/Dinodia Photos: 8; Jit Lim: 17. **The Bridgeman Art Library**/
British Library, London, UK 16t; British Museum, London, UK 14b. **Getty**/
Clicknique: 6; Stephanie Hager – HagerPhoto: 18T; The India Today Group
/ Contributor: 18B; Tatiana Kolesnikova: 35; Mike Timo: 15B; Westend61:
25; Caroline Woodham: 36. **iStock**/Clicknique: 9; fizkes: 37; iconogen-
ic: 35; Visiofutura: 21. **Rex Features**/Associated Newspapers/REX/
Shutterstock: 19T. **Shutterstock**/Bule Sky Studio: 13; claires: 213;
fizkes: 28, 216; f9photos: 205; Patrick Foto: 209; Evgeny Glazunov: 67;
GlebStock: 30T; Yekaterina Gurina: 23; Guschenkova: 30B; Olex Kmet:
58T; ostill: 2, 20; Photobac: 31; ppart: 14T; Yuriy Rudyy: 203; Lena
Serditov: 15T; thipjang: 42T; wavebreakmedia: 11, 16B.

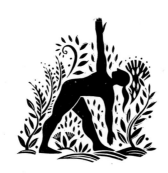